Forever Young

Reenita Malhotra Hora is schooled in Ayurveda, India's tradition of wellbeing, and is a consultant to prestigious spas throughout the USA, Asia and Europe. Her work as an Ayurveda educator has taken her everywhere, from California Pacific Medical Center and UC San Francisco School of Medicine to the pages of *Yoga Journal*. Born in Mumbai, she now lives in Hong Kong.

Forever Young

Unleashing the Magic of Ayurveda

REENITA MALHOTRA HORA

MACMILLAN

First published in the Indian subcontinent 2013 by Macmillan
an imprint of Pan Macmillan, a division of Macmillan Publishers Limited
Pan Macmillan, 20 New Wharf Road, London N1 9RR
Basingstoke and Oxford
Associated companies throughout the world
www.panmacmillan.com

ISBN 978-93-82616-02-3
Copyright © Reenita Malhotra Hora 2013

Typeset by Jojy Philip, New Delhi 110 015
Printed and bound in India by Thomson Press India Ltd.

For Pushpa Vij, who will always be forever young

Yaa Devi Sarvabhuteshu Vidyaroopena Sanstitha
Namastasyai Namstasyai Namastasyai Namo Namah

My respects to the Goddess who
exists in life as Knowledge
— *Markandeya Purana*

Contents

Foreword

Ayurveda is a 5000-year-old system of medicine that has much to offer anyone in search of a healthy lifestyle today. The Sanskrit word 'Ayurveda' has two roots: 'ayur', meaning 'life' and 'veda', meaning 'knowledge'. The systematic collection of health and healing knowledge encompassing all aspects of life and daily living has led the practice of Ayurveda to be called the 'science of life'. A comprehensive approach, Ayurveda includes concepts of creation and energy, precepts of the moral and ethical life and recommended practices relating to nutrition, physical activity, rest, relaxation and spiritual practice. It is truly a timeless practice based on centuries of careful observation and interpretation.

In *Forever Young*, Reenita Malhotra Hora gives us a guide to the practice of Ayurveda that yokes ancient wisdom

– both knowledge and practice – with contemporary reality. She understands the challenges of modern life and provides facts and routines that are understandable, accessible and doable. She teaches that true wellbeing and beauty originate within – they cannot be achieved through anything that covers or masks who we truly are. When we feel good, we look good. Feeling good requires a commitment to what we take in (in the form of food and drink, sounds, sights); what we feel (in the form of emotions and sensations); and how we relate to everything around us. Ayurveda is about balance, relatedness, lifelong learning and daily practice.

Forever Young, with its time-tested approaches, practical recommendations and straightforward language, is an invaluable book for all those open to taking responsibility for their own wellbeing.

WILLIAM B. STEWART, MD
Medical Director
Institute for Health and Healing
California Pacific Medical Center
San Francisco, California, USA

Introduction

I grew up in Bombay – India's most dynamic city, but also a place steeped in ancient traditions of the oldest living culture known. This contrast was also borne out in my own family, who expected that I would be educated in business and accounting before finding my place as the daughter-in-law of a Punjabi business family. I surprised my family and perhaps disappointed them by being a little too independent than they had taught me to be when I insisted on attending college in the United States. I was set on becoming a marketing professional of some sort. I saw myself as a completely modern woman.

Ayurveda was the furthest thing from my mind when I embarked on this educational adventure. After all, I had grown up with its ancient health traditions in the household. It was routine to me to practise yoga, eat chyawanprash with parathas at breakfast or oil my hair before showering. But something happened when I went to college. In an atmosphere of intense competition and high expectations, I watched many of my friends survive on a never-ending cycle of caffeine and Tylenol. Rather than listening to the demands of their own bodies, as I had been taught to do, they were trying to override their need for sleep and for good nutrition by using synthetic solutions. And it wasn't working – they told me over and over that they felt tired, stressed out, depleted. They looked it too. In fact, living life in overdrive has been aging people in the Western world well before their time. It was then that I began to realize how important Ayurveda is

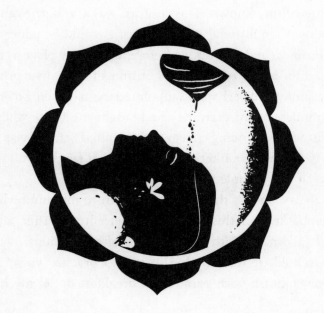

for health, for beauty and for longevity, and that I had lived all my life taking the ancient wisdom for granted. So I surprised my family again by deciding to pursue a career in Ayurveda. After I finished college, I decided to study Ayurveda, which in India is labelled the 'poor man's medicine'. I knew I would become a health educator and consultant, and, above all, an ambassador for this wonderful, ancient life science that was so much a part of me and the life that all of us in India lead.

I often ask myself how I got to this point. How did I come to this crossroads of so-called modern life and the ancient traditions of Ayurveda? The answer is my family. My late grandfather, Gopal Krishan Vij, left an indelible imprint on my life and values. He was a man who lived simply and sought to achieve his full potential in whatever task he took on, from being a civil engineer to being a father. He encouraged the women in his family to be strong and smart and achieve whatever they set out to do. Along with my grandmother Pushpa, he taught us all the subtle principles of Ayurveda, so that our minds and bodies would always be healthy. My grandfather also discouraged us from vanity and self-indulgence, from devoting our energies to jewellery, make-up and fashion – he knew there was more to life than that.

Under my grandfather's influence, the women of my family defined beauty not as something exterior, like a beautiful dress or sparkling jewels, but rather radiance that comes from health, confidence and self-esteem. My grandfather would often describe to me his mother, my great-grandmother, who woke early every morning to care for her family and dressed simply in a white sari, her clean skin reflecting the rays of the morning light: to him she was the embodiment of this ideal. It was because of her simple practice of Ayurvedic self-care that she not only lived a long life but remained youthful, energetic and radiant to the end of her days. Learning from her example, that kind of beauty became my ideal too. In writing *Forever Young*, my goal is to teach you the principles of Ayurveda so you can cultivate the same radiance, wellbeing and longevity that the women of my family demonstrated to me.

The following pages are designed to enable you to achieve inner beauty and longevity through a balanced, healthy, Ayurvedic lifestyle. This is a book for anyone who wants to end the cycle of stress and exhaustion and the toll this takes on our health and appearance by making simple, sensible lifestyle changes. *Forever Young* is an introduction to the principles of Ayurveda, and details how to put them to work. In Chapter 1, you will learn about the philosophy of Ayurveda and how it has evolved from an ancient medicine into a staple of the contemporary Indian household. You will learn about ojas – the life-force or vitality that is the source of inner beauty – and the science behind Ayurveda. Chapter 2 introduces the doshas – the 3 mind-body energies that are a part of each of us. You will learn how to determine which dosha is dominant in you, the key to selecting the yoga routines that will help you feel balanced and healthy. Chapter 3 offers recipes for traditional homemade cleansers and moisturizers for the hair, skin and body that are customized for your dosha, like a soothing milk and rice water bath (p. 58) or an exfoliating cleanser made from herbs you probably already have in your kitchen (pp. 34-37). Chapter 4 teaches you a balanced approach to fitness, focusing on yoga, which shares its origins with Ayurveda. You will learn how to choose a style of yoga practice that is right for you and the routines that are best for your body type. In Chapter 5, you will learn the principles of Ayurvedic nutrition and how to make smart choices. Chapter 6 describes seasonal practices for wellbeing, such as an at-home 'detox retreat', that will help you recharge your batteries. The last chapter is a guide to professional body treatments that will enhance your practice of Ayurveda.

Forever Young is not only an introduction to household Ayurveda, but also a potential tool for maximizing our longevity by restoring a sense of balance and sanity that is so often missing from our busy lives. The treatments and routines in this book are meant to help you be your best, feel your best and look your best – in short, to optimize the radiant youthfulness that you already have, now and forever.

ONE

What is Ayurveda?

Ayurveda is believed to be the oldest medical science in existence. Sanskrit for the 'science of life', it is a set of self-care guidelines that will help any person stay healthy and feel good by understanding the needs of his or her own mind and body. Ayurveda is intended to help each person be her best self – healthy, happy and radiant with beauty. Ayurvedic beauty treatments include skincare, diet, massage and exercise routines that are customized for every person to reflect their unique needs.

Ayurveda recognizes that we are all different – that each of us has a unique mind and body. After all, we look and behave differently from one another, and we all have different reactions to everyday situations. Everything from the foods we eat to the emotions we experience affects

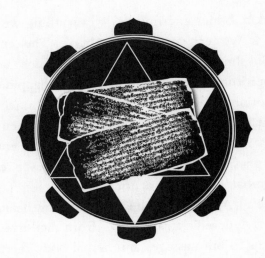

us each in our own way. We all have our own personal definition of what it means to be happy, healthy and in balance – that is, feeling full of energy and life. And because we are each unique, we all require different treatments and remedies to help us be our best. Ayurveda as a system includes tools to help figure out what these customized treatments should be.

Ayurveda acknowledges that the mind and body are not two separate entities but are closely intertwined. We have all seen how our thinking affects our body (say, when we are worried or upset and our skin breaks out) and how our body affects our mind (like the way our self-esteem plummets when we do not get regular exercise). Ayurveda has two special terms to convey this idea. The physical or tangible body, Sthoola Sharira, is our skin, bones and muscles – everything we would find in a Western anatomy textbook. The energetic body, Sukshna Sharira, is that with which we feel, sense, spiritualize, emote and think. So happiness and joy, emotional pain, psyche, perceptions, hunches and intuition are all considered to form part of our energetic anatomy. Ayurveda works on healing both the energetic and the physical bodies, because one can never reach its full potential if the other is not strong.

Above all, Ayurveda teaches us how to stay healthy and balanced. Ayurvedic treatments – from digestive herbal decoctions to oil massages and herbal body therapies – are intended to be gentle habits that can last a lifetime, not extreme regimes or quick fixes. Ayurveda is unlike many other health systems, which oversimplify the variety of factors that affect our health and how we feel and only address the symptoms, not the causes, of imbalance. Because many of us experience so much stress these days, and because 'feeling stressed' is really just another way of saying our life is out of balance, Ayurveda is more useful and important than ever before. It is the perfect antidote to stress because it addresses the whole person and how she is affected by her lifestyle.

THE ORIGINS OF AYURVEDA

Though its origins are lost to historians, Ayurveda is believed to have come from the Vedic gods over

5000 years ago, when a group of scholars and mystics met in the Himalayas to try to discover the secrets of longevity and the cures of illnesses of every kind. Through meditation and spiritual communion with the gods, the scholars and mystics arrived upon guidance for everything from everyday wellbeing to internal medicine and surgery. Ayurveda was an oral tradition in India for hundreds of years until it was collected into 3 main texts: the *Charaka Samhita*, the *Sushruta Samhita* and the *Ashtanga Hridayam*. The exact dates of authorship are not known, but the *Charaka Samhita* and the *Sushruta Samhita* are thought to have been written in the first few centuries BCE, with the *Ashtanga Hridayam* coming later, about 4900 CE. Together they form the basic compendia for Ayurvedic medicine today.

The essence of the medicine has also been captured in thousands of household traditions, some of which were incorporated into written manuscripts, and others that have simply been passed down as oral tradition. Many of the written manuscripts still exist as 'secrets of a traditional household'; others were lost over time but the oral traditions remain ingrained into the psyche of the modern Indian way of living. While household manuscripts are often written in the vernacular, the 3 main books are written in Sanskrit verse (Sanskrit is the ancient language of India, just as Latin is of the Western world). This vivid poetry articulates Ayurvedic philosophies and concepts. For this reason, it is hard to define whether Ayurveda is an art or a science. It might well in fact be both, as the Sanskrit verses reflect both on the theoretical aspects of Ayurveda – the art side – and the practical knowledge involved in incorporating it into daily life.

Traditionally, most Indian villages had their own Ayurvedic doctor who would advise the community about self-care practices and gather medicinal plants from the surrounding forests. This doctor would explain the meanings of the Ayurvedic sutras, or teachings, to student apprentices, who then prepared and dispensed medicines according to his instructions. In the years when India was a colony of the British Empire, the ruling powers tried to stop the practice of Ayurveda (amongst other traditional medicines) and it temporarily lost the cultural influence it once held. But after India became an independent nation in 1947, Ayurveda began to undergo a renaissance, and has since become popular all over the world.

Even today, Ayurveda is a part of everyday life in many Indian households without them even realizing it. For example, families drink water that has been stored in a copper vessel because Ayurveda recognizes that copper detoxifies the body and boosts the immune system. The sacred tulsi (basil plant), offered in prayer to the Indian god Vishnu, is typically placed in the central area of Indian homes to clarify the mind of impure thoughts and rid the environment of microbes. Finally, herbal kitchen remedies form a natural part of every Indian housewife's repertoire: common culinary items like turmeric, ginger and malai (dairy cream) are used for cooking, beauty treatments and to treat minor ailments.

OJAS: THE FOUNDATION OF INNER BEAUTY

Ayurveda teaches that health and beauty are the results of a powerful energy within us; the more of it we have in us, the better we look and feel. Maximizing this energy is the essential goal of Ayurveda. This energy is called ojas (pronounced oh-jus), which means 'that which invigorates'. It is the life-force, the energy that flows through every person and living thing. Like *Ch'i* in Chinese philosophy, ojas is the force that makes us feel happy and alive. Responsible for wellness, harmony and spiritual growth, it makes our eyes shine and puts a spring in our step. A high level of ojas brings bliss and happiness, which people around us see as radiance.

Ojas connects people and living things and is present in every aspect of life, from our emotional wellbeing to the foods we eat. For example, soil with strong ojas is rich in nutrients. It has the capacity to nurture a healthy apple tree that will root itself deep in the ground and grow to a substantial height. Filled with a high level of ojas, this tree bears lush, nutritious fruit. A woman who eats the fruit absorbs not only vitamins, but ojas, which provides her, both mind and body, with strength and longevity. When her own ojas potential is maximized, she is energized, inspiring everyone around her. The wheel turns full circle when the apple core goes into the compost heap and is recycled back into the environment, feeding the soil that gave life to the original tree.

When our ojas is low we are like dried leaves – tired, worn out, brittle. We experience a breakdown in the normal functions of the mind-body system and become susceptible to illness, both emotional and physical. The best way to keep our ojas up is to live a balanced lifestyle that is pure and close to nature. An overactive lifestyle (rajas) or a dull, inert lifestyle (tamas) both cause stress and deplete ojas. We must strive for a state of purity and balance, a third way of life called sattwa. Ayurvedic routines for personal care, both on a daily basis (dinacharya) and seasonally (ritucharya), help us stay in balance. Inner beauty will unfold naturally if you protect the mind and body against unhealthy influences and live in harmony with the natural laws of the universe.

DOSHAS: THE BUILDING BLOCKS OF BALANCE

We know that living in balance is the way to achieving and maintaining high ojas, the ultimate destination of our Ayurvedic journey. But what does it mean to live in balance? Ayurveda teaches that each of us is a unique individual, in how we think, move, act, how we react to stress, in the foods we like to eat, in the activities we enjoy. So balance would mean something different for each person. Ayurveda can help you determine the make-up of your mind and body – your natural tendencies and preferences. With this knowledge, it is simple to learn what to do (and what not to do) to even out those characteristics and achieve balance.

Ayurveda tells us that each person, like the world itself, is composed of 5 elements: space, air, fire, water and earth. The qualities of these elements are apparent in our physical bodies and our energetic bodies. For example, the light and mobile quality of air gives us the ability both to move our bodies and to be flexible in our thinking. The smooth and liquid quality of water gives sheen to our hair and makes for a nurturing disposition. But these 5 elements do not exist separately within us. Instead, they unite to form 3 distinct energetic forces called doshas. Each dosha is a combination of 2 of these 5 elements, and all are present to some degree in each person.

Air, which provides movement and space, which provides vastness, unites to form the vata dosha, which has an overall light, cold, dry and dispersing quality. Vata initiates movement in the mind – thoughts, ideas and creativity – and also physical movement, impulses in the nervous system, blood and lymphatic circulation, walking and even gesturing with the hands.

Fire, which provides heat and water, which provides fluidity, unites to form the pitta dosha, which has an overall heating, oily, sharp and penetrating quality. Pitta controls transformations in the mind such as intelligence, reasoning, passion and the operation of the senses, as well as physical transformations such as metabolism, hormonal activity, enzymatic behaviour and body temperature.

Water, together with earth, which provides solidity, unites to form the kapha dosha, which has an overall heavy, cold, oily and cohesive property. Kapha provides nurturing and lubrication to the mind and helps preserve the memory. It also binds and lubricates the physical tissues with mucus, body fluids and plasma, making the body stable and firm.

A proportion of each of these doshas in a person defines her prakruti, or mind-body constitution. Understanding your prakruti is like knowing how to read the blueprint for your own health, although a complete understanding of your prakruti is gained through meeting with an experienced Ayurvedic professional. In the next chapter you will learn more about prakruti, the 3 doshas and how to get a sense of what your own dominant dosha might be, which is the first step towards Ayurvedic healing.

TWO

Know Your Dosha, Know Yourself

The Ayurvedic concept of prakruti, which translates literally from Sanskrit as 'nature', refers to our mind-body constitution – the unique characteristics each of us is born with, perceptible through emotions, behaviour, body type, metabolism and health tendencies. The overall nature of a person's constitution is largely determined by which of the doshas (vata, pitta or kapha) is predominant. All 3 doshas exist in varying levels in each of us. Imagine a pie chart with three sections – the proportions are different for each person, but always add up to 100 per cent.

Most of us have a prakruti that comprises more of 1 dosha than the other 2. Our emotional capacity, physical

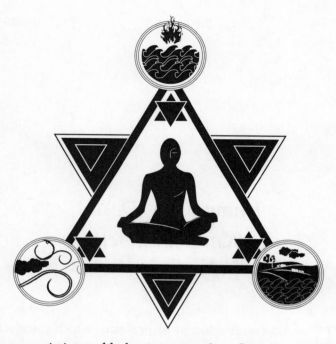

characteristics and behaviour mostly reflect the qualities of our dominant dosha. Some of us exhibit more than one of the dosha characteristics, in that 2 of the 3 doshas exist more or less equally in a higher proportion relative to the third. These are 'mixed-dosha' types. It is quite common, for example, to be a vata-pitta type, exhibiting the physical and emotional characteristics of both doshas. In other cases, one dosha might dominate physical traits and another show itself in emotional traits, or both characteristics could be a mix of both doshas. Very few people actually have equal proportions of all 3 doshas. For the purposes of this book, you will identify the one predominant dosha that characterizes your mind and body and will learn what to do to keep that dosha in balance.

To increase ojas, our core energy, we need to constantly harmonize our prakruti, our essential nature. So understanding prakruti and the elements that compose it becomes the natural first step in our journey to cultivate inner beauty. While everybody is born with a basic prakruti that is unique and will stay constant through life, the day-to-day interplay of dosha tendencies is likely to vary based upon influences from food, lifestyle, environment and seasons. We can examine our lifestyle to see whether we are 'living right' and maintaining harmony in our lifestyle, or whether our lifestyle is driving any of our doshas into excess. Once this happens, we can begin to use the diet, skincare regimen and fitness programmes or yoga techniques that work best to keep our doshas in balance.

As prakruti varies from individual to individual, so does the definition of balance. As stated earlier, according to Ayurveda, balance does not mean 'all things being equal' or all of us having equal amounts of each dosha within us. Instead, it is a state of equilibrium where our current dosha levels match the specific proportions of our natural mind-body make-up. When in equilibrium, the doshas help us be our best selves. But when they become aggravated, they create problems such as sluggishness, dehydration, inflammation and other sensitivities. If you consider that 'dosha' literally translates from Sanskrit as 'fault', it becomes clear that maintaining the equilibrium of the doshas is a challenge for us all, especially given the demands of modern living.

When first introduced to the concept, many ask the question: Which of the doshas is the best? In fact, they are all the best when they are in harmony, and they are all the worst when they are imbalanced. No matter what our dosha, the goal is to bring it into equilibrium and live closest to prakruti, our natural state of inner beauty.

VATA

The characteristics of vata (vayu = air and akash = space) can be likened to those of a desert or outer space – a vast amount of space with air moving through it. Unobstructed, the air can change its course with complete freedom and flexibility. People with a vata-dominant prakruti are creative and free-spirited. They have amazing power of thought and sometimes a bent towards spirituality. They make talented artists, composers, writers or scientists. Saraswati, Vedic goddess of knowledge, personifies the inner beauty of the vata dosha. She is the consort of Brahma, creator of the universe, and represents learning, creativity, knowledge and vitality of the intellect. In mythology she is always depicted holding a veena (wind instrument), a book and a beaded necklace, each bead representing a branch of ancient Vedic knowledge. Physically, vatas tend to be small-boned, with a tendency towards dry, thinner skin;

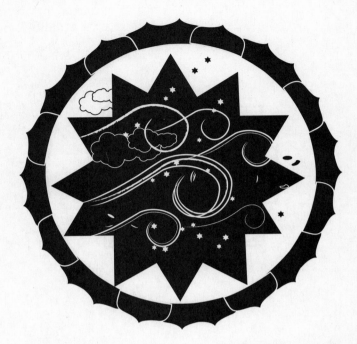

drier, more brittle hair; cold extremities; and erratic eating patterns, behaviour and habits. Vata doshas might have a hard time sitting still.

PITTA

The pitta constitution (tejas = fire and jal = water) is like a volcano – it has a liquid heat smouldering deep inside, which sometimes accumulates and comes rushing out with dynamic intensity and drive. People with a pitta-dominant prakruti are intense, organized and execution-oriented, with a fantastic sense of purpose. They are able

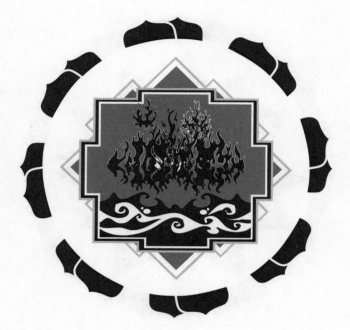

to process thoughts in a logical manner and make excellent leaders, managers or mathematicians. Parvati (Durga) is the goddess of strength and power and well represents the beauty of the pitta dosha, which can at once be destructive and dangerous as well as powerful and seductive. She is the consort of Shiva, the destroyer of negativity, and is his counterpart in providing humanity with the power of active energy to choose good over evil, and so maximizes ojas. Physically, pittas tend to have oily skin and hair with a 'patchy' quality to it (this can mean an uneven skin tone, combination skin that is more oily in the T-zone, thinner hair, and/or a certain flush to the skin). Their hair and skin react easily to hormonal sensitivity and they are generally more prone to feeling hot and irritable.

KAPHA

The soothing and stable qualities of kapha (jal = water and prithvi = earth) resemble those of clay – sand and water coming together to form something that can take shape and create vessels that have holding power without being easily disturbed. People with a kapha-dominated prakruti are nurturing, compassionate, meticulous and

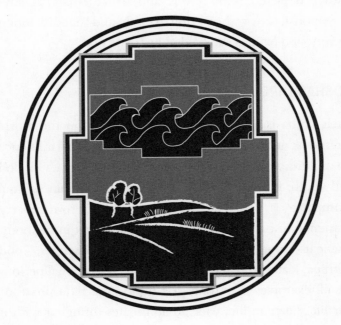

have a wonderful ability to put physical structure to ideas and plans. Such people make great healthcare workers, caregivers or workers in any occupation that requires persistence, physical stamina and precision. Physically, they are heavier, stable people with skin that is cool and moist to the touch, thick hair all over the body and thicker, spongier skin. Kaphas tend to feel cold and break out into cool, clammy perspiration. The kapha dosha is synonymous with bounty, especially that which lasts a long time. Lakshmi, goddess of wealth, exemplifies the beauty of the kapha dosha. The consort of Vishnu, the preserver of the universe, she is bountiful and earthy, always depicted with jewels and ornaments. Lakshmi is responsible for showering wealth and stability upon society, and exudes the golden lustre of ojas.

DOSHAS THROUGH LIFE

Each dosha is a type of energy that exists in the world around us, and each of these energies has a special influence on us during different stages of our lives. During childhood and youth, for example, kapha enhances chubbiness, so a plump baby is considered to have strong ojas. From puberty to menopause, pitta increases acidity and heat in the body, giving us strength to carry on through those changes. Good stamina, leadership and forbearance in transitional periods are all examples of strong ojas during the pitta phase of our life. Later in life, vata predominates, bringing with it wrinkles and drier skin, and challenges with digestion and sleeping. But this is also the time when our spiritual abilities are at their highest potential – it is the best time to develop a practice of meditation. Wisdom and spirituality are examples of strong ojas during this stage. Understanding your prakruti and how to increase your vitality will ensure that you look and feel your best at every stage of life.

DOSHAS OUT OF BALANCE

When doshas go into a state of imbalance or excess, we experience low ojas. Imbalances (vikruti) refer to an excess, or accumulation, of any one or more of the doshas, causing negative forces and toxins to begin spreading through the body. Minor excesses of vata, pitta or kapha are often manifested as dryness, a general sensation of heat and heaviness in the mind and body. We may become intolerant of foods with similar dosha qualities as our predominant dosha. Left unattended, these imbalances can develop into illnesses, so it is important to be aware of their symptoms.

The pressures of modern life wreak havoc with our doshas. In ancient times, people modelled their lifestyle on nature and the seasons. Today, environmental influences like light, heat and water that once ruled our work and sleep patterns are now under our control. Conveniences like eating seasonal fruit year-round, driving instead of walking and unhealthy diet and exercise habits distract us from our natural rhythms. As a result, it is easy to find ourselves feeling rundown, stressed and out of balance. Ayurveda recognizes the need to rejuvenate from within by setting the dosha composition back to prakruti, its natural starting point. This does not mean returning to the ways of our ancestors but, rather, gently adjusting our lifestyle to bring us back into balance.

Our predominant dosha is understandably the one most likely to become imbalanced. For example, vatas who are out of balance might have lower immunity and a tendency to catch colds on a regular basis. Each dosha expresses imbalance in a different way. Learning to read these signs will help you get back in balance quickly.

Vata is the most volatile of the 3 doshas. Too much vata energy creates dryness in the colon, causing pain, fatigue and lowered immunity. It sets into the mind as anxiety, fear and an inability to focus. People with vata imbalance tend to be 'spacey' and forgetful. They lack the ability to focus and behave erratically. Low skin elasticity begins to manifest as wrinkles. This is exacerbated by delicate nerves and disturbed sleep patterns. Pitta imbalances raise heat in the mid-digestive tract. Too much pitta energy manifests itself emotionally as anger, intolerance and criticism or physically as acidity, inflammation and sensitivities. People with pitta imbalances are prone to acne, heat toxins, any kind of '-itis, food sensitivities (or allergies), cosmetics, dust and pollen.

Kapha imbalances cause secretion of excess juices in the upper digestive tract, causing sluggishness, depression, water retention, fat and excessive mucus. People with too much kapha energy have clogged pores and follicles, mousy, congested skin and manifest 'couch-potato' behaviour – they are lethargic and eat for comfort.

The Dosha Quiz

This quiz will help give you a sense of your dominant dosha. While an Ayurvedic doctor can most accurately determine your prakruti, this quiz will help you identify your primary dosha, the building block of your self-care routine. For each question, choose as many answers as you feel apply to you. All your answers do not have to be from the same dosha type. Rather than trying to answer based on how you feel right now, or want to look and feel, think specifically about how you usually look and feel. Whichever dosha you answer with the most often is your predominant dosha. Keep this dosha in mind as you read about the routines for personal care, yoga and diet in the following chapters. While each of the doshas can go out of balance at any time, it is your dominant dosha that best predicts how you naturally feel.

The skin on my face is …

vata   normal to dry. I have a tendency towards fine lines and wrinkles. My skin lacks muscle tone or elasticity. It feels dry or tight when I travel, get dehydrated or go out in cold weather.

pitta   oily in the T-zone and dry on the cheeks. My skin tends to be sensitive and might redden or break out when exposed to chemicals, cosmetics, soap and synthetics. I might have moles, freckles or hyper-pigmentation.

kapha   normal to oily. My skin tone is quite supple and elastic, although my face might get puffy. I have a tendency to have large pores and sometimes get whiteheads and pustules.

The skin on my body is ...

vata   normal to dry. It is thin and translucent, so you can often see my veins through the skin. It can lack elasticity and sag in some places. It might be rough or flake easily in certain areas.

pitta   normal to sensitive. It is warm, has a flush to it and reddens easily, especially in the sun or warmer weather. It might scar easily or have hyper-pigmentation marks. I may scratch my skin in response to sensitivities, which then causes the skin to scar.

kapha   normal, thick and spongy. It has good, strong, supple tone and elasticity. My skin might retain water from time to time.

The temperature of my skin is ...

vata   cool or cold. I have cold hands and feet, and I usually feel cold, especially in dry weather.

pitta   warm. My skin is warm to the touch, especially in the upper torso, and my hands, feet, groin and underarms tend to perspire. I feel hot and sweaty fairly readily, especially in warmer weather. My perspiration can have an offensive odour.

kapha   cold. My skin might feel cool to the touch even in fatty areas such as the buttocks, hips, thighs and upper arms. It does not breathe well in cool, damp climates, and my pores tend to become clogged with oil. I often experience a cool, 'clammy-all-over' kind of perspiration.

My body frame is ...

vata   small, lean or wiry, either tall and thin or small and petite. I have lighter and less dense bones.

pitta   compact, athletic and muscular. I have a medium build and quite well-defined musculature and bone structure.

kapha   large. I have wide hips and shoulders. I have large muscles, and dense and heavy bones.

My body frame has ...

vata   less amounts of fat right under the skin. I can lose (or gain) weight quickly and can get 'scrawny' at times.

pitta   a medium layer of fat right under the skin (more in some areas and less in others). I have a good, strong metabolism and can gain or lose weight relatively easily.

kapha   a thick layer of fat under the skin. I can gain weight easily, and find it relatively hard to lose weight.

Without chemical treatments, the texture of my hair is …

vata   wavy, dry with a flyaway tendency. My scalp tends to be dry and may flake when rubbed. I sometimes have dry, scaly dandruff.

pitta   fine, oilier in patches. My scalp can be sensitive to chemicals in hair products and prone to dandruff.

kapha   lustrous, beautiful with natural shine and moisture. My scalp can be slightly oily to the touch. Sometimes the oil can clump up, forming large, oily flakes of dandruff.

The strength and thickness of my hair is …

vata   inconsistent. While each individual hair might be thin and relatively dry or brittle, I have a lot of hair on my head.

pitta   fine. Each individual hair is fine; the overall volume is thin and can even seem scanty. I am prone to premature hair loss or greying hair.

kapha   thick. Each individual hair is strong, thick and resistant to damage. I have lots of hair on my head.

My nails are ...

vata   normal to dry. They break easily and are better managed if kept short. They might have ridges.

pitta   pinkish and fairly strong.

kapha   big and thick with prominent white moons. They are strong and resistant to damage.

My eyes are ...

vata   small with sparse lashes. They get dry easily.

pitta   sharp and clear. They are sensitive to bright light and redden easily with external influences like dust, pollen, cosmetics, strong light or foods that do not agree with me.

kapha   large and picturesque, perhaps even dreamy. They might get puffy or have some whitish discharge from time to time.

My digestion is ...

vata   irregular. Sometimes I am hungry at mealtimes and sometimes I am not. I might forget to eat and then feel spacey or weak, or tend towards constipation, gas, bad breath and hard, dry or small, rabbit-like stool.

pitta   intense. If I delay eating past my regular
         mealtimes, I get irritable. I sometimes get loose
         stool, heartburn or acidity. My stool can be
         'explosive'.

kapha   consistent or low. I can go without a meal if I am
         still full from the last one, but I also tend to eat for
         comfort. I often have a slower passage of thick,
         well-formed stool, perhaps lined with mucus. I
         might even go a day or two between stools.

My sleep pattern is ...

vata   light and interrupted. I might stay awake for part
         of the night or have fitful, interrupted sleep. I
         usually cannot remember my dreams, but when
         I do they tend to be vivid or imaginative.

pitta   regular. I sleep about the same number of hours
         and feel rested. I have active dreams, sometimes
         even violent ones.

kapha   deep and heavy. I sleep long hours. I am not a
         morning person.

Emotionally speaking, I am ...

vata   quick-minded, creative and imaginative. I am
         perceptive, excitable and can get restless. I am
         friendly and exuberant.

pitta   an organized and disciplined person. I am usually
         quite intense and passionate about what I do.

kapha   calm, steady and nurturing. I do not get easily influenced or excited. I am a loyal, loving friend.

Intellectually speaking, I am ...

vata   all over the place. I sometimes find it difficult to focus because I get excited about things. I tend to have a short memory.

pitta   sharp, analytical, intelligent and focused. I have a good memory, and good management and leadership skills.

kapha   slower to catch on to things. I learn by doing and repetition. I have a long-term memory.

When I manifest emotional imbalances, I...

vata   become anxious, stressed, nervous or fearful. I might get spacey or find it hard to focus when I am stressed.

pitta   become critical, controlling and angry. I range from being irritable to completely volatile when I am stressed.

kapha   become stubborn and stuck. I hold things in, 'shut down' and become impossible to communicate with when I am stressed.

The pace of my life is ...

vata   intentionally fast. I keep myself busy to stay happy and prevent boredom.

pitta   intense. My activities are well laid out and organized but require my absolute focus and involvement.

kapha   slow. I like to follow through my personal projects at my own pace.

AYURVEDIC PANTRY

In the chapters that follow, the recommendations and recipes for self-care call for a number of ingredients, some common, some perhaps less so and some that are probably completely new to you. This chart lists the staples of any Ayurvedic pantry and explains their significant properties for Ayurvedic practices. As you learn more about your dosha and the imbalances you tend to experience, you will find yourself customizing this list to meet your personal needs.

Ayurvedic herbal ingredients are available through Ayurvedic shops, natural-food stores and mail-order suppliers (see *Resources*). Shop in places where you know the stock is turned over frequently, and use fresh herbs or whole-leaf dried herbs whenever possible. Dried herbs begin to lose their effectiveness after about 6 months, even sooner when ground, so buy only a little at a time. Some of these ingredients can be found in compounds such as vata tea, pitta tea or kapha oil, so keep a lookout for them as you shop around.

OILS AND GHEE

coconut (nariyal) oil

This cooling oil is ideal for balancing pitta. Used as both a hair and body oil, either alone or enhanced with medicinal herbs and flowers.

ghee

Known in culinary terms as clarified butter, this is an ideal moisturizer for vata, as it is extremely penetrating, and pitta, as it is sweet and cooling. It is important to use ghee that has been prepared in the traditional style and not a big brand that has been processed like commercial butter. See also p. 75.

mustard oil

This healing oil is ideal for kapha. A common ingredient in cooking, it can be used as a moisturizer or in bath water and ubtan (skin scrub).

neem oil

This anti-inflammatory and anti-septic oil is wonderful for cuts, abrasions, insect bites and allergic reactions.

sesame (til) oil

This warming, nutritious oil is suitable for all three doshas, and particularly for vata. It is used both in cooking and as a body moisturizer infused with medicinal herbs and flowers.

MEDICINAL HERBS

amla
: This fruit has a high content of Vitamin C and is full of antioxidants. It increases ojas in all tissues and is powerful for balancing pitta in the blood cells and tissues.

brahmi
: Translated as 'divine creative energy', this rejuvenating herb, known to calm and cool the mind, is ideal for balancing pitta and vata. It is believed to promote intelligence and eternal youth and can be used in teas, salads and hair oils.

dashmool
: Meaning '10 valuables' in English, it is a mixture containing the roots of 10 key medicinal herbs. Ideal as an herb tea, this is a powerful ally in the flu season.

neem
: The antiseptic quality of this bitter herb, celebrated for its blood-detoxifying and skin-healing properties, makes it an extremely effective ingredient in cosmetics,

medicines, pharmaceuticals and even tooth powders. It is used in ubtans to balance both pitta and kapha.

chandan (sandalwood)	A pitta-balancing essential, it is used to rejuvenate and cool the skin. Applied to the forehead, it takes the edge off headaches.
triphala	The 3 fruits – amalaki, bhibhitaki and haritaki – comprised in this mix balance each of the 3 doshas and cleanse the entire digestive system. Key to seasonal detoxifying programmes, triphala may be taken everyday – as a tea with milk, or mixed with honey or ghee.
tulsi	This plant, known as the 'holy' basil, has properties that aid in building immunity and preventing illness. Used in ubtans, in bath water, as an herb for tea and in face packs, it is an invaluable ingredient in skincare. Look for the fresh version at your local farmers' market, or purchase a plant for your home.
haldi (turmeric)	A powerful blood purifier, this common cooking spice is also a boon to ubtan formulas. Be careful

to use only a small amount, as its colour is quite penetrating and can stain the skin.

OTHER FOODS AND PLANTS

kumari (aloe)
A cooling plant that grows in hot desert terrain, this pitta-balancing gel is ideal both as a moisturizer and as a juice mix.

chana besan
Also known as gram flour, this chickpea flour product is the perfect ubtan base. Use with turmeric root, sandalwood, tulsi and other dried herbs to remove excess oil and cleanse the skin.

cucumber
Cooling and moisturizing, cucumber is excellent for ubtans and moisturizers. Also use to cool hot, tired eyes.

ginger
An important Ayurvedic ingredient, this vata- and kapha-balancing root is useful for teas, oils and food flavouring.

malai (cream)
Highly nutritious and moisturizing, this is the perfect vata-balancing food for the mind, body and skin.

madhu (honey)	A natural sweetener, ideal for tempering the challenging tastes of Ayurvedic medicinal herbs. As a humectant, it can also be added to any of the moisturizer recipes and is particularly ideal for vata cleansers.
jasmine	Used for infusing in massage oils and bath water for vata and pitta, the many varieties of this flower are quite fragrant. If the flower is not available, an essential oil will do just as well.
gulab jal (rose water)	An ideal toner for all skin types; also an effective and gentle eye wash.
yogurt	Wonderful for balancing the pH of the skin, this is a widely used ingredient in ubtans and moisturizers.

THREE

Household Beauty Traditions
Skin, Hair and Eye Care

Ayurveda emphasizes beauty from within, beauty that comes from health and wellbeing, not from cosmetics or anything that tries to cover up the true you. Because healthy skin and beauty go hand in hand, Indian women are encouraged to care for their complexion from a very young age. Simple, all-natural beauty treatments that emphasize balance and serenity have been passed down by Indian women from generation to generation. These easy routines for caring for your skin, hands, feet, hair and eyes all help to balance the doshas and increase vitality or ojas.

Since your face and body reflect your health and your feelings, the best way to look your best is to feel your best,

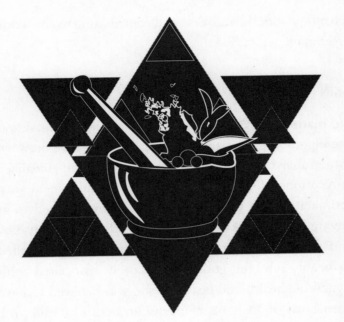

by taking time out for yourself every day. The Ayurvedic daily routine (dinacharya) is composed of a few simple rituals designed primarily to make you feel good. The daily regimen is as much a mindset as it is a list of practices, and includes waking up early to maximize the day, cleansing, bathing, exercise and a soothing, self-applied oil massage. Following these rituals can allow you a few moments in the day to focus inward, quiet your mind and focus on appreciating the gift of health. While many of us feel we do not have much time to take care of ourselves beyond a quick shower, Ayurveda tells us that tending to our mind and body with care is the starting point for living in harmony with the universe and contributing to the world around us.

SKIN

No matter how many times we hear or read that skin is the biggest organ, many of us hang somewhere between forgetfulness and despair about our skin. Idealized perceptions of beautiful skin abound and can in turn intimidate; even the Vedic goddesses are referred to as having beautiful skin that has the radiance of sunshine and the smoothness of silk. Lakshmi, often described as beauty's bright goddess, is closely associated with Ayurvedic health and beauty – she was believed to have been born of Vishnu's churning an ocean of milk. For us mortals, Ayurveda teaches daily and weekly skincare practices to make the skin glow with inner and outer health. These practices focus on not only cleaning and protecting the skin but also stimulating and cleansing the blood and the lymph, the 2 primary fluids that directly feed the skin.

The dosha skin types chart below will help you better understand your skin. Look for treatments appropriate to your skin type throughout this section. If your skin feels normal, use any treatments for your dosha that appeal to you. If your skin feels unhealthy or shows signs of imbalance, enlist those treatments that target the problem: if dryness is your issue, for instance, focus on moisturizing treatments that balance vata. You will also find self-massage techniques, simple bath soaks and shower scrubs for overall balance.

Dosha Skin Types

Although by now you should have a good idea about which elements, or doshas, dominate in your constitution from taking the quiz in the previous chapter, it is worth taking a closer look at your skin specifically to see if it reflects one particular dosha. Regardless of skin type, many of us experience fluctuations in the mood of our skin from day to day and season to season. The following lists will help you determine your Ayurvedic skin type, what sensitivities to be aware of and what signs of imbalance to watch out for.

vata	
complexion	normal to dry, with a slightly rough texture
colouring	pale and thin, almost translucent, with veins sometimes showing through
pores	small, fine
sensitivities	sensitive to changes in climate; tendency towards chapping and dryness
aging	loses elasticity; tendency to sag and develop wrinkles and/or stretch marks

imbalance	excessive dryness or chapping (lips and skin); wrinkles or dark circles under the eyes, cellulite or stretched skin around the buttocks and thighs; peeling skin on feet and around toenails; corns and calluses
pitta	
complexion	combination, oilier in the T-zone and drier on the cheeks; perhaps slightly moist or oily to the touch
colouring	warm, soft with strong colouring
pores	fine, with larger pores in the T-zone
sensitivities	sunburns easily, bruises easily and tends to develop freckles, moles or spider veins; sensitive to chemicals; tendency towards blackheads and collecting sweat and dirt
aging	becomes sensitive with age and prone to hot flashes
imbalance	excessive flushing, inflammation, acne, rosacea, hyper-pigmentation; cold sores; athlete's foot or other fungal infections; easy scarring

kapha	
complexion	moist or oily to the touch; well toned, spongy or thick
colouring	cool, soft, with even colouring
pores	large all over
sensitivities	holds oil; tendency towards whiteheads and clogged pores
aging	ages well, with consistent tone and minimal wrinkling
imbalance	swelling, water retention; clogged pores, whiteheads; puffy eyes; fatty lumps on the body; clammy hands, excessive oil and perspiration

ABHYANGA: OIL APPLICATION

Ayurvedic skincare begins with abhyanga, a therapeutic self-applied oil massage that nourishes the skin. Because looking good depends on feeling good, giving yourself a massage everyday may be the best beauty secret you can utilize. The combination of the gentle motion of the massage and the healing power of herb-infused oils is optimum for stimulating the dosha energies to carry on their natural functions and retain balance, as well as for toning the skin and its underlying muscles and tissue. The

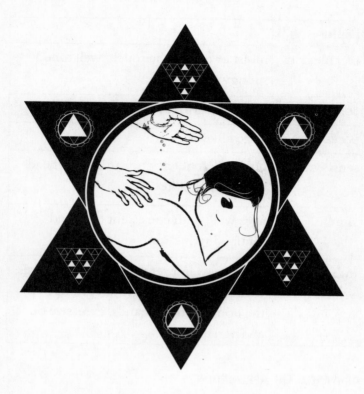

infused oils used for massage have rejuvenating properties
that we miss out on if we think of all oils as impurities
(like grease and dirt) or as sources of automatic acne or
other breakouts, since the right oils actually help remove
toxins. Though Ayurvedic herbal extracts are available
in creams, oils are much more effective moisturizers.
Besides, Ayurveda believes that every day of abhyanga,
the medicinal oils penetrate each of our 7 tissue layers
successively. This is why professional Ayurvedic centres

typically recommend abhyanga massage over a course of 7 (or multiples of 7) days.

If using oils feels strange to you, start practising abhyanga with an unprocessed oil like coconut or sesame. Using an unprocessed oil is critical even though it might be more 'sticky' or odiferous than a refined, processed oil. The latter is typically made for the cosmetics industry but has virtually no ability to grab on to toxic matter in the tissue layers. Once you have chosen your oil, focus on the soothing effects of the massage. Abhyanga is traditionally a daily massage for the face and entire body, but if you do not have enough time for the full routine, focus on the head, face, hands and feet for optimum results.

Abhyanga massage is traditionally performed with oils prepared from medicinal herbs that balance the doshas. If you are feeling healthy, use the oil for your dosha, otherwise use the oil for the dosha that is out of balance (i.e., if your skin is irritated, use a pitta oil). While these herb-infused oils are available from specialty shops and from the resources listed towards the end of this book, it is also easy to make your own simple, infused oil by combining a base oil with readily available culinary herbs, spices and flowers, many of which you might already have in your own kitchen. These oils will moisturize your skin gloriously while the scent will transport you, and the massage you give yourself will give you time to focus inward everyday. Here are some recipes for making your own Ayurvedic abhyanga oils. See the Ayurvedic Pantry (pp. 32-37) for more information on the ingredients used here.

Abhyanga Massage Oils
(Makes 1 cup)

 VATA ABHYANGA OIL

1 cup ghee or sesame base oil

¼ cup mixed herbs; fresh (or dried if this not available) turmeric root, fresh ginger, lotus root, fresh cloves and fresh orange peel, jatamansi, jasmine or rose flower petals, ashwagandha root powder in any combination*

Essential oils (optional): jasmine, basil, orange, rose

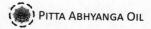 PITTA ABHYANGA OIL

1 cup ghee, coconut or sunflower base oil

¼ cup mixed herbs: fresh (or dried if this not available) turmeric root, camphor pieces, manjistha, neem, shatavari, white sandalwood in any combination*

Essential oils (optional): pine, sandalwood, tea tree/neem

 KAPHA ABHYANGA OIL

1 cup sesame base oil

¼ cup mixed herbs: fresh (or dried if this not available)

turmeric root, tulsi, fresh ginger, fresh lemon peel,
cardamom and cloves, in any combination*

Essential oils (optional): patchouli, eucalyptus, rosemary

🌿 In a small saucepan, heat the oil gently until it is beginning
to boil but not smoking.

🌿 Stir in the herbs and remove from heat.

🌿 Cover and let the herbs steep in the oil for 1 day or up to
2 days. Strain the oil through a coffee filter or a double
layer of cheesecloth into an airtight container.

🌿 Add 5-8 drops of single or mixed essential oil, if desired.

Notes

*Although for the purposes of this book I have stipulated precise measurements, the traditional Indian household goes by the concept of 'andaaze se' (go with the amount you think it should be). So rather than getting bogged down by the recipe, treat it more as a 'formula'. It is perfectly fine to add more of one ingredient and less of another or to substitute an ingredient that you cannot find with something else.

If you do not want to prepare your own facial abhyanga oil but prefer to buy something readymade, then look for these at your local Ayurvedic shop: **vata**: jatamansi, jasmine or rose oil; **pitta**: shatavari oil, neem oil, plain ghee or coconut oil; **kapha**: ginger oil or plain sesame oil.

Specialty stores like Forest Essentials offer a variety of readymade abhyanga oils:

vata: Cold-Pressed Body Massage Oil Indian Rose & Geranium, Cold-Pressed Body Massage Oil Madurai Jasmine & Mogra

pitta: Ayurvedic Body Massage Oil Balaswagandha

kapha: Cold-Pressed Body Massage Oil Lime & Ginger

FULL-BODY ABHYANGA MASSAGE

Ayurvedic abhyanga is traditionally done prior to bathing. Ideally, every morning you would spend 5-10 minutes on the massage routine, rest for about 15 minutes, then shower with a natural cleanser or non-detergent soap. If you do not have enough time in the mornings, apply the oil lightly following your shower, or aim to do it at night, after you shower and before you go to sleep.

Abhyanga works from the centre of the body outward to the extremities. This follows the natural energy pattern, regulating tissue metabolism and providing for maximum distribution of ojas. Movements are either linear, following the layout of the muscles, or circular, applied typically to the joints, scalp and vital energy points such as the navel. Linear movements encourage the natural flow of vata energy throughout the physical and emotional body; circular movements help release energy in areas where it can become 'stuck', leading to pitta or kapha imbalance. Heat your massage oil bain-marie style in a small bowl over warm water, or keep it at room temperature.

¼ to ½ cup abhyanga massage oil of your choice, homemade (pp. 46-47) or purchased

Pour a little oil onto the crown of your head and gently massage this area to help stimulate the release of heat and negative energy. Apply oil lightly and evenly all over the head and massage from the hairline to the crown, moving in small circles. Massage up and down the back of your neck. Massage in front of your ears, then behind, then your earlobes.

Rub your shoulders in small circles, then massage in straight lines from the neck outward to the shoulders. Massage from the centre of the chest over the breastbone and out to the shoulders, then from the area where the ribs meet out to the periphery along and under the rib cage.

Placing one hand over the other, use the bottom hand to massage your navel in a small, clockwise circle (in the direction of the colon), gradually increasing the size of the circle. Using both hands together (or placing one hand over the other for greater pressure), massage the front of your body from the navel to the left side of your waist, and up over your breast to the shoulder. Repeat on the other side, again using both hands. Use both hands to massage your waist from back to front.

Using the opposite hand, massage one shoulder in straight strokes down to the elbow and onto the hand. Rub the elbow and wrist in circles. Switch arms and repeat. Rub one palm then the top of the hand. Pull and rotate each finger in succession. Massage the base of each finger. Switch hands and repeat.

Massage in straight strokes, as far as you can reach, from your lower back upward. Use your left hand to massage the right shoulder blade up to the shoulder. Switch arms and repeat. Massage your hips and buttocks in outward circles, starting small and increasing the size of the circle as you go.

Massage the front and back of your thighs in straight strokes to the knees. Rub your knees in small, circular movements. Massage your calves from the knees to the ankles and back. Massage the ankles in vigorous, circular strokes. Massage the tops of your feet and the webs of your toes. Pull and rotate each toe in turn. Massage the balls of your feet. Rub the sole of one foot with the palm of the opposing hand to create friction. Repeat with the other foot.

ABHYANGA OF THE FACE AND NECK

Massaging your face and neck moisturizes the skin and also helps the abhyanga oils to penetrate. Your massage movements should be applied upward, towards the temples, like a natural face lift.

2 to 3 tablespoons abhyanga oil of your choice, homemade (pp. 46-47) or purchased, warmed to room temperature if necessary

Apply oil lightly from the bridge of your nose over the cheeks and out to the ears. Rub your temples in small circles, then massage in circles up the hairline. Rub from the centre of your eyebrows upward and outward over your forehead. Use 3 fingers of either hand to massage in circles all over your forehead.

Using both hands, massage in straight strokes from the centre of your upper lip outward under the cheekbones to the ears. Using the index finger of each hand, rub over and around the inside edge and then outside your nostrils in circular movements. Then use 3 fingers of each hand to massage in straight strokes outward from your nostrils to your ears. Massage in front of and around your ears. Massage your earlobes and inside the ears.

Apply gentle pressure on your cheekbones in an upward direction towards your temples. Pinch-press along the eyebrows, starting at the centre of the brow and moving outward. Press on your eye sockets by closing your eyes and patting from the inside corners to the outside.

Starting with your fingers under your jaw, manipulate the area from your jawline to the base of your neck in a piano-playing motion, with gentle but firm pressure.

BODY CLEANSING (UBTAN)

In the Ayurvedic skincare routine, abhyanga is followed by ubtan, a form of cleansing with therapeutic massage. Ubtan uses cleansing pastes prepared from herbs and flours or coarsely ground legumes. These clarify the skin by drawing heat from the blood and stimulating lymph flow and also exfoliate the skin and firm up the body. Traditional ubtan pastes use medicinal herbs such as manjistha, neem and sandalwood (see pp. 53-55) that break down congested toxins in the blood and lymph and encourage the body to shed toxins naturally. Babies are traditionally rubbed down with an ubtan paste at birth to cleanse them of impurities and strengthen their co-ordination.

Ubtan cleansers can be applied either as pastes or powders, and are rubbed into the face and body fairly vigorously to stimulate the release of toxins. Vata types should use a more liquid application with relatively large, circular movements – their skin being fine, powders can be a little too abrasive. Pitta types benefit from a smooth paste application that can be easily worked in circular movements without over-stimulating the skin. Kapha types require a powder application and should use small, vigorous, vibratory circular movements to really stimulate the natural flow of body fluids. Remember that you can use the ubtan recipe for your dosha, or the ubtan recipe for the dosha imbalance you are experiencing.

Ubtan cleansers are available in Ayurvedic shops but here are some simple recipes for making your own. Make sure facial cleansers are ground smoothly enough to not irritate your skin. These may be used for the body as well. Because the skin of the body is less delicate than that of the face and neck, any cleanser used for the body can be coarser and used with a little more vigour to help tighten the pores and invigorate the underlying muscle and lymph tissue. When cleansing your body, if you have time, apply the ubtan paste, leave it on for 10-15 minutes until it begins to dry and then rub it off. See the Ayurvedic Pantry (pp. 32-37) for more information on the ingredients used here.

Facial Ubtans
(Makes 1 application)

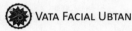 VATA FACIAL UBTAN

Vata types benefit from a more liquid ubtan that warms and moisturizes the skin.

5-6 raw, blanched almonds, skin removed

¼ cup malai (cream)

2 tablespoons sesame oil

1 teaspoon finely ground brahmi or tulsi (see pp. 34-35)

- In a bowl, soak the almonds in the cream overnight.
- In a food processor, combine the almonds with the cream, sesame oil and herb. Pulse until the mixture is smooth but yet has plenty of texture.
- Rub into your face using gentle, circular motions. Let the ubtan soak in/dry for 5-10 minutes. Dust off excess.
- Rinse off with cool to lukewarm water if necessary.*

* Traditionally, ubtans are not washed off. The excess is dusted off and the ingredients left to be absorbed into the skin through the day. If, however, you cannot handle this then feel free to wash off the excess traces of the ubtan.

If you prefer a readymade ubtan, try Tejasvi Milk Facial Ubtan, a completely natural skin wash and pack containing red sandalwood, wild turmeric, saffron, manjistha, fig leaves and jivanthi, all of which even the skin tone and add lustre. Or try Roop Nikhar & Gulab Facial Ubtan, a fresh rose petal-and-almond-based formulation for porcelain-smooth, glowing skin.

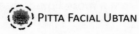 PITTA FACIAL UBTAN

This pitta ubtan paste cools the skin and extracts heat toxins.

3 teaspoons chana besan

¼ teaspoon ground turmeric

2 teaspoons ground white sandalwood or
½ teaspoon sandalwood essential oil

2 tablespoons crushed cucumber

- In a bowl, stir together all the ingredients.
- Rub the mixture into your face using small, circular motions. Let the ubtan soak in/dry for 5-10 minutes. Dust off excess.
- Rinse with cool water if necessary.

For a readymade version, try Soundarya Facial Ubtan, an ancient recipe comprising 52 herbs including turmeric, fennel seeds, star anise fruit, lemon, orange, sandalwood, fenugreek, manjistha, cinnamon, nutgrass tubers, clove, nutmeg, marigold, marjoram, poppy seeds, camphor and saffron, all of which leave the complexion soft, glowing and gently polished.

 KAPHA FACIAL UBTAN

Kapha types benefit from a powdered ubtan that stimulates the skin to reduce water and accommodates natural lymph flow.

3 teaspoons mung dal

1 teaspoon fenugreek seeds

1 teaspoon ground, dried orange peel

1 teaspoon Ayurvedic herbs such as
neem powder (see p. 34), long pepper (pippali)

- With a mortar and pestle, crush all the ingredients, taking care to break up the mung dal into small pieces.
- Rub the mixture into your face using small, vigorous circular movements. Let the ubtan soak in/dry for 5-10 minutes. Dust off excess.
- Rinse with cold water if necessary.

For a readymade version, try Multani Mitti Facial Ubtan, an ideal treatment for blemished skin made of alkaline clay, jadhikai, sandalwood and green gram powder. Its deep-cleansing action unclogs pores, lifts excess oil and impurities and purifies the skin, leaving it clean and fresh.

Ubtan Body Scrub for any Dosha
(Makes 1 full body application)

Here is a good, all-purpose tri-dosha ubtan recipe for the whole body. Apply following your daily self-massage. Leave on for 10-15 minutes before rinsing, if you have time. Follow this with a light application of abhyanga oil to moisturize further.

1 cup chana besan

½ teaspoon ground turmeric

2 tablespoon ground mustard

3 tablespoons rose water

❀ For vata dosha, in a bowl combine all the ingredients with ½ to ⅔ cup of ghee (see pp. 75-76) and stir to blend; the mixture should be a relatively liquid paste. Smooth into the skin with gentle, circular movements, then rinse off with warm water.

❀ For pitta dosha, in a bowl combine all the ingredients with ½ cup fresh kumari (aloe vera) pulp and ½ cup coconut water and stir to blend. Work into the skin vigorously but without over-stimulating it.

❀ For kapha dosha, in a bowl combine all the ingredients with 1 cup yogurt and stir to blend; the mixture should be a relatively coarse paste. Work into wet skin vigorously then rinse with warm water.

For something different, you could try Body Polisher Hydrating Sea Salt Crystal Rose and Body Polisher Cane

Sugar & Tamarind which incorporate natural, mineral-rich sea salts and raw, unprocessed cane sugar to buff the skin along with pure cold-pressed almonds and apricot oils to provide hydration.

BATHING

In India, bathing represents a cleansing not only of the physical body but also of the spiritual self. Many purification rituals are associated with bathing; it is believed that ritual bathing in the waters of the River Ganga will purify the soul. In a simple Ayurvedic context, a bath taken in the morning following self-massage (see p. 43) is likened to bathing in the Ganga.

In addition to cleansing body and spirit, bathing is associated with numerous other benefits to the mind and body. The *Ashtanga Hridayam*, one of the ancient Ayurvedic texts, tells us that bathing improves sleep, appetite, sexual vigour, life span and enthusiasm. The royal queens and princesses in ancient India were bathed in milk and fresh herbs to moisturize their skin until it glowed. To this day in India, special ingredients are stirred into a hot bath to customize it taking into account dosha, time of year and/or other considerations. For example, in the north, mustard is added to bath water in the winter months for a warm dip that balances kapha dosha, which can become aggravated in the late winter and early spring.

Bathing rituals are also believed to significantly impact health, especially over the long term. For example, warm water is believed to strengthen the body, while the face and head should be rinsed in cool water, as this is the area that naturally releases heat. Applying hot water to the head is believed to disturb the release of heat from the crown, weakening the hair roots and encouraging emotional irritability and 'hot-headedness'. So, while you can relax in a warm shower or bath, remember to wash your hair and face with cool water. Try the recipe below for your dosha for a balancing herbal cleansing bath. Remember that you can use the bath recipe for your dosha, or the one appropriate to any imbalance you are feeling. The mixture can also be made with a little water or ground into a paste for use as a shower scrub.

BATHS

✹ Vata Milk and Rice Water Bath

The tradition of bathing in milk was begun by queens and noblewomen in ancient India. Milk contains proteins that are vital for nourishing the skin, and rice starch softens the skin and relieves stress. In a bowl, mix 1 cup powdered milk with 1 cup rice starch. Stir in 2 tablespoons of rose water for fragrance and softness. Dissolve the paste in your bath or in your balti if you are accustomed to bathing with a balti and mug.

Pitta Fresh Herb and Flower Bath

A herb and flower bath is perfect for soothing easily irritated pitta. You will be naturally perfumed with the fragrance of a Vedic garden. This is especially good in summertime, when pitta influence is at its peak. Add ½ cup marigold, rose or jasmine flower petals and a handful of cooling fresh herbs such as mint or coriander to your bath water or balti. Adding a couple of tablespoons of lemon juice or white vinegar would help balance excess oil and get rid of blemishes.

Kapha Mustard and Fenugreek Bath

This combination of herbs is traditional in the cold winter and winter monsoon season of the Punjab region. Use year-round but especially during the late winter and through spring, when kapha influence is at its peak. Add 3 tablespoons ground mustard and 1 tablespoon fenugreek powder to your bath or in your balti if you are accustomed to bathing with a balti and mug.

MOISTURIZING

Moisturizing the skin is extremely important to alleviate drying vata tendencies and to maintain suppleness and elasticity. The use of natural foods, botanicals and oils is the traditional Ayurvedic approach to nourishing and replenishing the skin. Moisturizing the face and neck can be done in the morning or evening, but is a must for your everyday routine (dinacharya). (Moisturizing the entire body is undertaken once a week.) Vata types with drier skin would do well to moisturize the face and neck twice a day, whereas pitta and kapha types can get away with moisturizing just once a day.

Here you will find moisturizer recipes for each dosha; remember that you can use the recipe for your dosha, or one that matches any imbalance you are experiencing. Since Ayurvedic moisturizers are made from natural ingredients that can grow bacteria, they do not keep too long. Prepare enough to last a few days at a time – ½ to 1 cup – and store in a cool, dry place. Avoid refrigerating the moisturizers as this will disrupt the natural chemistry with your skin in relation to the weather or outside temperature.

Moisturizers

 VATA

Vata skin needs plenty of natural moisture and oil to keep it supple and maintain elasticity. Ghee (see pp. 75-76) is the best moisturizer base for vata skin. In a bowl, mix together equal parts ghee and rose water. Add a teaspoon of honey and a few drops of your favourite essential oil to impart fragrance. Transfer to a jar with a tight-fitting lid. Rub a small amount of the solution onto your face and neck at least once a day. This recipe makes for an ideal moisturizer for both day and night applications for vata skin types. Sesame oil may be substituted for ghee.

 PITTA

Pitta skin needs a light moisturizer that is also cooling. Aloe is an ideal ingredient for both moisture and the wonderful soothing sensation it brings. For a daytime moisturizer, in a bowl combine 1 part brewed liquorice tea, 1 part aloe vera gel and 2 parts coconut or sunflower oil. Use the moisturizer on your face and neck at least once a day. At night, moisturize with equal parts aloe and ghee, or just plain ghee.

 KAPHA

Kapha skin is generally well toned and needs only a mild, balancing moisturizer. Pure mustard oil is an ideal base. In a bowl, mix together equal parts mustard oil and almond oil. Add a few drops of your favourite essential oil to dissipate the smell of mustard. This moisturizer is ideal for head-to-toe use, both day and night, but if the faint smell of mustard during the day bothers you, almond or sunflower oils are good alternatives for kapha skin.

A number of readymade moisturizers are available at Forest Essentials stores across India and online for the different dosha skin types:

vata: Sanjeevani Beauty Elixir and Tejasvi Night Emulsion Treatment (ghee-based)

pitta: Sanjeevani Beauty Elixir, Eternal Youth Formula Date & Litchi and Tejasvi Night Emulsion Treatment

kapha: Panchpushp Replenishing Light Moisturising Facial Gel or Pure Rosewater Light Hydrating Facial Gel

The build-up of toxins and wastes in the system, along with exposure to ultraviolet radiation and chemical air pollutants, slows down the regeneration of new cells. Research by Forest Essentials has revealed that gold actually helps transport oxygen molecules directly into the skin, influencing cellular functions and reversing damage by oxidation.

Using a gold-based facial serum is the perfect way to get added nutrients into deeper layers of the skin and speed up cellular regeneration. Try their serum prepared with natural oils and herbs and gold bhasma or ash such as Advanced Soundarya Age Defying Facial Serum.

WEEKLY SKINCARE RITUALS

Beyond your daily skincare regimen, it is a good idea to establish a weekly skincare ritual – a guaranteed timeout will truly work to beautify from within. While the guidelines outlined previously address your 'must-do' self-care for dinacharya, you need to go a little beyond this to really work at pulling out the toxins and maintaining balance for maximum ojas through the year. Traditionally, many of these beauty routines were followed as part of a daily detox and self-care programme but these days, our busy schedules and work or family commitments do not allow for deeper self-care or an everyday basis, so it is practical to seek out a routine that can be performed at least once a week. Try the weekly ritual ideal for your dosha described here, or switch to those for other doshas when you are feeling an imbalance. The most important part of the experience is to focus inward and tune into the needs of your dosha. As you incorporate weekly cleansing into your lifestyle, you should, over the weeks, begin to perceive a positive difference in your emotional being as you work from the angle of your physical being. See the Ayurvedic Pantry (pp. 32-37) for more information on the ingredients used here.

Weekly Cleansing Mask

 ### Vata Weekly Cleansing Mask

1 teaspoon honey

1 teaspoon rose water

1 cup plus 2 teaspoons malai

- ❧ Following self-massage (see p. 45), prepare a mask by whisking together the eggwhite, honey, rose water and 2 teaspoons malai in a bowl. Set aside.
- ❧ Prepare a steam bath by turning on a hot shower and letting it run for a few minutes until it begins to generate

steam. Point the shower head away from you so that you can step into the shower cubicle to immerse yourself in the steam but without actually getting wet from the running water, if possible, or clear a space outside the shower where steam is accumulating. Remove all of your clothing and enter the steamy area, closing the shower curtain or door, if applicable, so that the steam does not escape. Find a place to sit if there is not a natural perch – if there is room, position a chair in the space. Relax in the steam bath for about 10 minutes. Turn off the shower.

❧ Apply the mask to your face and neck. Step into the shower area if you are not already there and leave the mask on for 15 minutes while rubbing the cup of malai all over your body. You should be able to stay warm from all the steam that has been generated.

❧ Rinse your face and body thoroughly; your skin will feel soft and supple.

PITTA WEEKLY CLEANSING MASK

2 teaspoons sandalwood powder

1 pinch of ground turmeric

1 teaspoon neem oil (see p. 33)

2 tablespoons multani mitti or natural clay
(available at health-food stores)

¼ cup fresh orange juice

1 cucumber, peeled and coarsely crushed

2 teaspoons ground neem (see p. 34) or fresh coriander
leaves or seeds

🌿 Following self-massage (see p. 43), prepare a mask by
stirring together the sandalwood, turmeric, neem oil,
clay and orange juice. Set aside.

🌿 Separately, stir together the cucumber and ground neem
or coriander. Prepare a steam bath by turning on a hot
shower and letting it run for a few minutes until it begins
to generate steam. Point the shower head away from you
so that you can step into the shower cubicle to immerse
yourself in the steam but without actually getting wet from
the running water, if possible, or clear a space outside the
shower where steam is accumulating. Remove all of your
clothing and enter the steamy area, closing the shower
curtain or door, if applicable, so that the steam does not
escape. Find a place to sit if there is not a natural perch –
if there is room, position a chair in the space. Relax in the
steam bath for about 5 minutes. Turn off the shower.

🌿 Apply the mask to your face and neck. Step into the
shower area if you are not already there and leave the
mask on for 15 minutes while rubbing the cucumber
mixture all over your body.

🌿 Rinse your face and body thoroughly; your skin will feel
deeply cleansed and moisturized.

 KAPHA WEEKLY CLEANSING MASK

2 teaspoons ground neem (see p. 34)
1 pinch of ground turmeric

4 tablespoons ginger juice

1 cup yogurt

2 tablespoons salt

2 tablespoons ground black pepper

❧ Following self-massage (see p. 43), prepare a mask by stirring together the ground neem, turmeric, clay and ginger juice. Set aside.

❧ Prepare a steam bath by turning on a hot shower and letting it run for a few minutes until it begins to generate steam. Point the shower head away from you so that you can step into the shower cubicle to immerse yourself in the steam but without actually getting wet from the running water, if possible, or clear a space outside the shower where steam is accumulating. Remove all of your clothing and enter the steamy area, closing the shower curtain or door, if applicable, so that the steam does not escape. Find a place to sit if there is not a natural perch – if there is room, position a chair in the space.

❧ Apply the mask to your face and neck. Step into the shower area if you are not already there and leave the mask on for 15 minutes while rubbing the yogurt mixture all over your body. You should be able to stay warm from the steam that has been generated.

❧ Rinse your face and body; your skin will feel toned and detoxified.

vata: Madhulika Nourishing Honey Lep by Forest Essentials is a nutritious facial paste made from raw organic honey mixed with nourishing herbs, flowers and fruit. Use it after cleansing and toning your skin.

pitta: FE Facial Treatment Masque Nourishing Mysore Sandalwood & Nagkesar is a nourishing face pack made with pure sandalwood, rosewater, black Himalayan clay and potent herbs. Make a paste of this with fresh orange juice.

kapha: Yogurt is a most nutritious food. FE Facial Treatment Masque Purifying Natrural Yogurt contains Ayurvedic herbs and extracts to cleanse, purify and nourish the skin. Narangi & Nagkesar Facial Ubtan can be mixed with yogurt to use on the skin.

HANDS AND FEET

Bathing and care for your hands and feet deserve a special note. Ayurveda honours the hands and feet, and considers them magnets that attract life energy. Vedic goddesses are portrayed with multiple arms and hands holding symbolic objects or positioned in poses called mudras that instil divine energy. Walking barefoot is thought to draw energy from the earth. Washing and massaging the hands and feet everyday is therefore an essential part of Ayurvedic self-care. Massaging the hands and feet boosts circulation, helping alleviate vata problems like dryness or cold extremities, as well as kapha problems such as water retention.

The hands and feet reveal much about any dosha imbalances you are suffering. Use the chart below to identify constitutional imbalances, and read on for the solutions that are best for you.

vata	wrinkled or rough hands rough, hard feet nails that break or peel easily or have ridges cold hands and feet
pitta	fungus in the nails athlete's foot cuticles that bleed easily hot, sweaty hands and feet
kapha	puffy, swollen hands cold, clammy hands and feet thick layers of superfluous skin heavy, clumsy movement of the extremities

As a general practice, wash hands and feet with a mild soap, then massage with the appropriate Ayurvedic abhyanga oil to relieve dosha imbalances. Or, for simple, all-purpose moisturizing, use sesame oil or ghee (see p. 33).

Once a week, give your hands and feet a balancing treatment with a special scrub and moisturizer. You will be amazed at how smooth and supple your skin feels, resonating with the vital energy of the earth.

Start by dipping the smooth side of a kasha katori (a

bowl made of an alloy of 5 metals: copper, tin, zinc, iron and mercury), rubbing it on the soles of your feet for about 5 minutes. By helping to draw out heat from the body, this procedure calms your nerves and detoxifes your skin. Follow this with an ubtan.

For vata and kapha imbalances, make a paste of 1 teaspoon rock salt, ½ teaspoon ground cloves and 2 tablespoons sesame oil. Rub the mixture in small circles into both hands and feet, focusing on the heels, soles, ankles, finger and toe webs, fingers and toes, wrists and palms.

For pitta tendencies, make a solution of 1 teaspoon neem oil (see p. 33) and 2 tablespoons sesame oil. Rub the mixture in small circles into both the hands and the feet, focusing on the heels, soles, ankles, finger and toe webs, fingers and toes, wrists and palms.

For an all-purpose treatment, rinse the hands and feet with the juice of 1 lemon diluted in a cup of warm water. Dry off with a soft, fluffy towel. Finish off by massaging 3-5 tablespoons of heavy whipping cream into your hands and feet to moisturize thoroughly.

HAIR

In India, hair symbolizes strength for men and beauty for women. It is believed that the Ganga was released to the Earth through Lord Shiva's tresses. Because of the belief that a significant amount of strength lies within the hair, Ayurveda prescribes everything possible to keep a cool head and maximize hair thickness. Internal heat is expelled through the top of the head, and higher levels of internal heat correspond to less hair, which is why pitta types tend to have thinner hair than kapha and vata types. Ayurvedic beauty rituals for the hair and scalp use cooling oils and other pitta-balancing herbs, fruit, nuts and flowers that focus on removing heat, strengthening hair follicles and promoting thickness. Yoga, pranayama and abhyanga techniques also focus on releasing heat through the crown.

Basic imbalances in the doshas can lead to problems of the hair and scalp. Vata imbalances (and also hairdryers) can cause dry, brittle or flyaway hair and dry dandruff. Pitta imbalances cause scalp sensitivity or premature greying and hair loss. Kapha imbalances dull the hair and scalp with excess oil secretions, which sometimes result in large flakes of oily dandruff.

Ayurvedic hair care is much gentler than that of the West. The hair is not washed everyday; daily cleansing strips the scalp of natural oils and encourages the sebaceous glands to produce more oil than necessary. Instead of washing the hair often and then using multiple products to restore shine and softness, hair is conditioned with oil prior to limited shampooing.

Begin your practice of Ayurvedic hair care by learning to brush your hair thoroughly everyday, and wash it only once or twice a week. (This can be hard to get used to at first, but you will soon find that washing your hair less frequently rebalances the flow of natural oils to your scalp, making it shiny and well-conditioned.) Then adopt the hair-care basics detailed below for strong and beautiful hair for any dosha.

ARITHA SHAMPOO
(Makes 1 application)

Aritha, the fruit of the soapnut tree, is extremely gentle and an effective agent for cleaning your hair without stripping the natural oils (though it does not lather like regular shampoo). Shikakai, another Ayurvedic botanical, provides additional conditioning.

> 1 cup whole aritha nuts or ½ cup aritha powder
>
> 2 tablespoons shikakai powder
>
> 1 tablespoon fresh lemon juice

❧ Soak the aritha in a cup of water overnight. (If using aritha powder, just stir into a cup of water and proceed with adding the lemon juice.) Strain the soaking liquid through a coffee filter or cheesecloth and add the shikakai powder and lemon juice. Apply the entire mixture to your hair (be careful not to get it get into your eyes as the aritha will sting) and rinse with cold water. It is best to let your hair air-dry, although you can blow-dry and style it as you are accustomed to, if necessary.

❧ If you are not inclined to prepare the aritha shampoo yourself then add 1 tablespoon all-purpose Ayurvedic hair oil or plain coconut oil to your regular shampoo for additional conditioning. Try to find as natural a shampoo as possible that minimizes the use of sulphates.

COCONUT AND FLOWER HAIR OIL
(Makes 1 application)

Oiling your hair is the most important part of Ayurvedic hair care. Not only does it beautify the hair and scalp, it helps reduce heat from the head, promoting sleep, relaxation and memory and increasing your all-round vitality or ojas. Use this basic oil to condition your hair before shampooing or, if you like, purchase the traditional Ayurvedic oils that contain bringh raj, brahmi or amla at an Ayurvedic store.

½ cup coconut oil

½ cup mixed fresh or dried flower petals such as red hibiscus (the latter is ideal as it helps prevent hair loss), marigold, rose or jasmine

- In a small saucepan, bring the oil to a boil. Reduce heat.
- Add the flowers, return to a boil and cook for 3 minutes.
- Remove from heat.
- Let the flowers steep in the oil for 1 day, then strain the oil through a coffee filter or a double layer of cheesecloth into an airtight container.
- To oil your hair, gently massage 4-5 tablespoons of the oil onto the crown of your head and into your scalp. Comb the oil out to the ends of the hair. You can apply a turban made of towel or plastic wrap so the oil really penetrates. Leave the oil in for at least 20 minutes, or overnight.

Forest Essentials offers plenty of sulphate-free shampoos and readymade hair oils specifically formulated for your dosha.

vata: Ayurvedic Herb Enriched Head Massage Oil Sugandha

pitta: Ayurvedic Herb Enriched Head Massage Oil Bringh Raj

kapha: Ayurvedic Herb Enriched Head Massage Oil Japapatti

EYES

In Indian tradition, eyes radiate powerful energy – look at any painting of the goddesses' almond-shaped eyes. Keeping the eyes healthy is the best way to keep their power at their peak, not to mention the best way to discourage dark circles, fine lines and red, itchy, watery eyes. The Ayurvedic approach to caring for the eye area is unique because it takes into account the eye itself; the skin around the eyes area is unique because it takes into account the eye itself, the skin around the eye and even how what you see affects you. Moisturizing your lids and caring for the surface of your eyeballs as well as gazing upon something beautiful are equally important ways of caring for your eye area.

The eyes are delicate and susceptible to various imbalances of the doshas. Sudden changes in temperature, straining, excessive crying, feeling angry, suppressing emotions, pollution and intoxicants all harm the eyes.

Vata imbalances dry out the eyes, causing wrinkles, lines, crow's feet and twitching eyelids. Pitta eyes can become itchy, red, heated and sensitive to light. Kapha imbalance leads to puffiness, swelling and sometimes excess secretion or glazed vision.

To keep your eyes healthy, wash them with cool water or rose water every morning, being sure to open your eyes for ablution. Once a week, apply 3-5 drops of ghee to the eyes to keep them cool. Or wash your eyes with ghee using an eyecup, filling the entire cup with ghee and placing it over one eye. Slowly open your eye to the ghee in the cup and blink and rotate the eyeball to bathe it completely. When you are done with the ghee eye bath or application of ghee drops, gently massage the skin under and around the eyes with a little more ghee or a few drops of heavy whipped cream. To complete the ritual, pinch the eyebrows from inside to outside and apply gentle pressure on the eye socket from inside to outside.

Kaajal – Protection against the Evil Eye

Kaajal has traditionally been used in the Ayurvedic beauty regime to soothe, cleanse and protect the eyes, both from infection and the proverbial evil eye. You can make your own kaajal though this traditional method from Kashmir.

In a clean glass vessel, prepare a solution of 100 ml

rose water and 5 grams of rasanjan (an extract from the barberry plant). Stir the solution for a few days then strain it. A few drops a day in the eyes clears up infection. Mix into the solution 2 teaspoons freshly ground turmeric power, 2 ground almonds and 2 dried and powdered nimbu (lime) leaves. Prepare a thick, flat roll of cotton wool, like a wick, and soak it in the mixture. Let the wick dry and twist it tightly. Place it in a flame-proof katori, preferably silver, filled with mustard oil or ghee. Light the wick and invert a second silver or earthenware cup over it about an inch from the flame.

Remove the upper cup 2 or 3 times as the wick burns and scrape out the soot (kaajal) into a pure silver container (silver is a cooling metal hence good for the eyes). Keep adding oil to the bottom cup till you gather as much kaajal as you require.

GHEE – THE LONGEVITY ENHANCER

Ghee, or clarified butter, is believed in Ayurveda to be one of the most sattwic foods, as it promotes memory, intelligence, agni (digestive fire) and ojas. Excellent for all 3 doshas, though specifically for vata and pitta, ghee is ideal for cooking as it has a high smoke point and does not burn easily. It provides nourishment to the body and builds healthy tissue when used in cooking, when taken alone or when prepared with medicinal herbs for skin, scalp and eye treatments. Ghee is also used for abhyanga.

Although ghee is readily available at Indian grocery stores, it is simple to make your own at home. I do not suggest making it from milk cream as the cream requires churning to turn it into butter. Although you can churn the cream with a mixer, I am not in favour of machine-churned butter as this upsets the natural cooling property of ghee.

You can, of course, make ghee from hand-churned organic butter. Clean and sterilize a saucepan by filling it with water, covering it with the lid and bringing it to boil for 30 minutes. Discard the water and add 1 pound unsalted organic hand-churned butter cut into chunks to the pan and put on low heat for 10-15 minutes, until the foam that collects on the surface begins to settle at the bottom of the pan. Continue to cook, stirring the top occasionally, until the ghee begins to boil gently. Remove from the heat and let it cool. Pour the clarified butter on top into a clean container, leaving the sediment at the bottom of the pan. As long as it is kept away from moisture and other contaminants, ghee keeps indefinitely without refrigeration because the milk fats that cause butter to spoil have been removed.

When ghee is at room temperature, it can be semi-solid, so run warm water over the closed container to soften it before using it for treatments.

FOUR

Yoga and Fitness

A tranquil mind and body, free of stress and tension, is the ultimate Ayurvedic beauty secret. Exercise creates vitality or ojas by releasing stress and building strength, flexibility and increased stamina. The results: glowing skin, a happy mood and a sense of serenity. While every kind of exercise has its particular benefits, yoga is the perfect complement to Ayurveda because its ultimate purpose is to regularize the flow of vital energy, or prana, in the system to increase ojas.

Yoga means 'union', as in that of the mind, body and breath. This integrated approach makes yoga very different from other forms of exercise. For example, instead of developing your voluntary muscles to their greatest capacity, yoga works with breath and movement

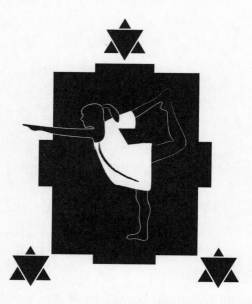

to help you gain control of your internal organs and
involuntary muscles. Instead of working the body to a
point where it needs to rest in order to rejuvenate and
strengthen itself, yoga invigorates the body by using
the breath in a way that creates inner strength and
stamina. In particular, the Ayurvedic approach to yoga
includes cleansing of the mind and thoughts in order to
detoxify the system – this is considered as important to
the workout as the arms and legs. Ayurveda encourages
various traditions of yoga, although the hatha yoga
tradition is the easiest to follow as a self-care technique.
An Ayurvedic approach to yoga goes beyond the physical
postures (asanas) to include meditative breathing
(pranayama), massage (abhyanga) and cleansing rituals

to awaken the body and control the subtle heating and cooling energies we experience in yoga.

Yoga and Ayurveda are sister disciplines. The original texts of yoga and Ayurveda were both believed to have been written by the snake bearer of Lord Vishnu, the preserver of the universe, during his earthly incarnation. In this context, 'preservation' means those actions that sustain and develop human life. Ayurveda and yoga both preserve the physical, emotional and spiritual body by simple self-care through daily life. Yoga believes that you are as young as you are flexible, and emphasizes the development of flexibility along with breath control to promote longevity. In fact, traditional Indian medicine does not necessarily consider yoga and Ayurveda to be two separate things.

YOGA STYLES

Many styles of yoga have developed over the last several years. The differences are in emphasis, such as focusing on strict alignment of the body, co-ordination of breath and movement, holding the postures or the flow from one posture to another. All of the styles share a common lineage and are based on Patanjali's *Yoga Sutras*, the classical yoga text of ancient India. No one style is 'better' than another, although certain styles can be favourable to particular doshas. Above all, it is important to find a style that you are comfortable with and a teacher who you can trust to improve your yoga practice.

HATHA

Hatha yoga is a classical style of yoga that is described in the *Yoga Sutras* and forms a base for many styles of yoga. It uses poses (asanas), breathing (pranayama) and relaxation to awaken, experience and control the subtle energies within. It provides strength and flexibility through a relatively gentle, inward experience.

ASHTANGA

Ashtanga means '8 limbs' in Sanskrit. These refer to the 8 limbs of yoga laid out in the *Yoga Sutras* of Patanjali. The Ashtanga method of asana practice was interpreted by T. Krishnamacharya and Sri K. Pattabhi Jois from an ancient text called the *Yoga Korunta*, which described as a unique system of hatha yoga developed by Vamana Rishi.

Ashtanga yoga is physically demanding. You flow through a series of poses, jumping from one posture to another to build strength, flexibility and stamina. The practice stresses breathing techniques (ujjayi breathing), locks (mula bandha and uddiyana bandha) and focus exercises (drishti).

SIVANANDA

Sivananda yoga follows the teachings of Swami Sivananda. The Sivananda ashram is situated in the sylvan surroundings of the Neyyar dam and forests just outside

Kerala's capital city, Trivandrum. The approach is holistic, offering yoga, devotion and philosophy.

INTEGRAL

Integral yoga was developed by Sri Swami Satchidananda who went to the US to teach yoga in the 1960s. The integral method seeks to integrate the mind, body and spirit by emphasizing breathing, meditation and kriyas (sequences) in addition to postures. This is a consciousness-oriented yoga that emphasizes healing and transformation. It is used by Dean Ornish in his ground-breaking work on reversing heart disease (1990).

IYENGAR

The Iyengar style of yoga was developed by B. K. S. Iyengar following his studies with his yoga guru Krishnamacharya in Mysore, in an effort to improve his health while suffering from tuberculosis.

It is one of the most popular styles of yoga in the world. Its great attention to detail and the precise alignment of postures is aided by the use of props such as blocks and belts. The sequences are systematized by level and can be gentle or challenging.

KRIPALU

Kripalu yoga is often called the 'yoga of consciousness'. It emphasizes proper breath, alignment and co-ordination of breath and movement, working according to the limits of your individual flexibility and strength. You learn to focus on the physical and psychological reactions caused by various postures to develop an awareness of mind, body, emotion and spirit.

KUNDALINI

Kundalini yoga is an ancient form of yoga that was popularized by Yogi Bhajan in the late 1960s. It focuses on the controlled release of kundalini, a powerful energy that is believed to be seated at the base of the spine. The practice involves classic poses, breath, co-ordination of breath and movement, and meditation to release this energy upward through the spine.

Yoga for your Dosha	
vata	Hatha, Bikram, Viniyoga, Kripalu
pitta	Iyengar, Viniyoga, Kundalini, Integral
kapha	Ashtanga, Bikram, Viniyoga, Kundalini

TRADITIONAL NASAL CLEANSING – JALNETI

The Ayurvedic tradition of jalneti is the act of cleansing the nasal passages with herb-infused water. Although it may seem hard or uncomfortable, with a little practice it is easy to do, and is highly effective. People suffering from allergies will particularly benefit from this practice, as cleansing the nasal passages with water and herbal oils purifies the system and helps regulate pressure in the head. It is best practised in the morning prior to breathing exercises such as pranayama. Jalneti is traditionally performed with a small pot called a neti pot that looks like a miniature teapot with a particularly long spout (see *Resources*). Fill the neti pot with 1 cup lukewarm water. Add 5-7 drops of an herbal essential oil that brings out toxins and relieves congestion (if these are not available, a teaspoon of table salt will help break down the upper levels of congestion). Place the spout at the right nostril (but do not insert into the nostril), keeping your mouth open to allow for free breathing, and the tip the pot to the left so that the water flushes through the nasal passages and emerges from your left nostril by the force of gravity. This will feel strange at first! Should any nasal congestion prevent the free flow of water, allow some time to elapse before trying again. When the pot is empty, refill and repeat with the other nostril. Work up to 2 pots per day on each side. Nasal cleansing is good for all 3 doshas.

YOGA DINACHARYA – YOGA RITUALS FOR EVERYDAY

While many treat yoga as an outlet for physical exercise, there is more to it than just the poses, or asanas. Without incorporating the other aspects of yoga, according to the ancient texts, it is nearly impossible to get the maximum benefits out of the physical postures. While you may feel like you do not have time enough to do a full practice all the time, start by making the time when you can: you may discover it is an easier habit to cultivate than you think. Even enjoyed only once in a while, yoga is a great restorative when you really need to take care of yourself. A complete yoga practice is ideally done in the morning, although it may be done in the evening as well.

A complete yoga practice has 5 parts. First, perform a simple self-massage (abhyanga), as described on p. 43. Second, try the nasal-cleansing routine to detoxify the system, as described on pp. 82-83. Third, using the guide below, develop a routine of yoga postures that are suited to your dosha-balancing objective, or attend your favourite yoga class. Fourth, end your asana practice by taking time for an exercise to control and focus the breath. Last, meditate on a favourite image, situation or positive thought.

YOGA TO BALANCE YOUR DOSHA

While working with an experienced yoga instructor is optimum for truly tailoring yoga to Ayurvedic needs, it is easy to incorporate dosha awareness into your practice at home. The following are simple yoga routines for each dosha that can help correct imbalance, or vikruti, on a day-to-day basis. Each sequence starts gently and builds in intensity as it goes along. Remember that you do not necessarily have to do the entire sequence everyday.

Depending on your dosha, your health on a particular day and your goals, your yoga can be a gentle, inward experience, or an athletic or aerobic practice.

VATA YOGA ROUTINE

Vata imbalances generally mean you are not feeling as strong as usual and that your immune system is more vulnerable to illness. Your metabolism fluctuates, resulting in chills, fatigue, emotional anxiety, stress, sleep disorders and even dry skin. Yoga routines that balance vata focus on stabilizing the tissues, grounding the body, calming the mind and enhancing strong bones and digestion.

The Easy Pose: Sukhasana

Sit on the floor (or on a cushion if this more comfortable), legs outstretched and wide apart. Draw in your right heel and anchor it at your crotch. Draw in your left foot and tuck it under your right leg. Keep your spine erect. Extend both arms so your palms rest on your knees. Breathe in and then slowly exhale. Repeat for 5-10 breaths.

Wind-free Pose: Pavanmukta Asana

Lie on your back with your legs together and arms by your sides, palms down. Bring your right knee to your chest, hugging it with both hands. Raise your chin towards your knee (or if that is too difficult, leave your head on the floor); keep your left leg relaxed. Breathe in and then slowly exhale. Hold for 5-10 breaths. Release and repeat on the other side. Then, contract your abdominal muscles to raise your legs about 6 inches off the floor. Raise both knees and hug them to your chest. Raise your chin towards your knees. If this is uncomfortable, keep your head on the floor. Breathe in and then slowly exhale. Hold the position for 5-10 breaths. Exhale completely and, holding the exhalation, contract your anus. Hold for a moment then relax the anal region. Release your legs with an inhalation. Repeat the sequence 2-4 times.

Warrior II Pose: Virabhadrasana

Stand straight with squared hips and feet 3-4 feet apart. Breathe in, raising your arms straight out to your sides at shoulder level. Exhale and turn your right foot, knee and leg to the right. Bend the right leg 90 degrees, keeping your chin perpendicular to the floor and your hips facing squarely forward. Keep your right knee over your right heel. Keep your left leg and knee straight but not locked and turn your left foot slightly inward. Lengthen your lower back, opening your chest forward and upward. Breathe in and then slowly exhale. Repeat for 5-10 rounds of breathing. Then slowly release. Repeat the pose on the other side. Repeat the entire sequence 2-4 times.

Stomach Lock: Uddiyana Bandha

Stand with squared hips and feet 3-4 feet apart. Bend your knees and squat, placing your hands on your knees, fingertips facing in. Inhale then exhale forcefully through an open mouth. Hold your breath, close your mouth and tuck your chin into your chest. Suck your abdominal muscles back, up and under your rib cage. Continue to hold the lock for 5-7 counts. Release your abdominal muscles. Inhaling, straighten your legs and come up to a stand. Exhaling, bend forward and hang loose. (Note that holding the breath is contraindicated for heart issues.)

Thunderbolt Pose: Vajrasana

Start by positioning yourself on your hands and knees, then sit back on your heels and look forward. Keep your spine straight and place your palms on your thighs near your knee joints. Breathe in and then slowly exhale. Hold the position for 5-10 breaths then exhale completely.

Cobra Pose: Bhujangasana

Lie face down. Position your legs together with the soles of your feet facing up and your forehead on the floor. Place your palms flat on the floor near your shoulders. Raise your head slowly, then the upper portion of your body to the pelvis (but keeping your pelvis on the floor). Arch your back as much as possible without placing pressure on your hands. Breathe in and then slowly exhale. Hold for 5-10 breaths, then release. Repeat 2-4 times.

Half Locust Pose: Shalabhasana

Lie face down, arms by your sides. Turn your chin towards but not touching the floor. Contracting the muscles of your waist and lower abdomen, raise your legs off the floor as high as possible (or raise one leg at a time if that is too difficult). Breathe in and then slowly exhale. Hold for 5-10 breaths, then release. Repeat 2-4 times.

Plough Pose: Halasana

Lie flat on your back, legs together. Raise your legs slowly up and over your head until your toes touch the floor. Keep your knees straight but not locked and the palms of your hands flat on the floor, arms outstretched. Take the hands towards the head and, interlocking the fingers, place the palms behind the scalp. If that is too difficult, use your hands to support your hips. Breathe in and then slowly exhale. Hold for 5-10 breaths, then release. Repeat 2-4 times.

Corpse Pose: Shavasana

Lie flat on your back with your arms at your sides, palms up and feet spread apart. Focus on your breath. Become aware of each part of your body and consciously relax it. Start with your right leg, working part by part from toes to groin, then relax your left leg in the same way. One at a time, relax your right and left hand and arm, working from fingers to shoulders. Then relax the front portion of your trunk, lower abdomen to upper abdomen, chest and throat. Then relax your back, from the lumbar region to mid-back, neck, face and the top of your head.

Meditative Breathing: Pranayama

This breathing exercise, called Suryabhedna, focuses on increasing heat in the body. Sit comfortably in a cross-legged position and slowly become aware of your breath. Take 10 natural breaths. Use your fingers to close your left nostril and inhale slowly through the right nostril. Retain your breath for as long as you comfortably can and then adjust your fingers to block the right nostril as you breathe out slowly through the left nostril. Build up breath-retention time with subsequent practice but only to a level of comfort, and never rush out-breath. 10-15 minutes of this pranayama everyday is extremely beneficial.

PITTA YOGA ROUTINE

Pitta imbalances are indicated by inflammation in the body and may manifest as excessive hunger, thirst and/or hypersensitivity, which may take the form of allergies, fevers or indigestion. Negative and angry moods may also result. Yoga routines that balance pitta focus on creating coolness and on cleansing impurities in the blood.

Stomach Lock: Uddiyana Bandha (see p. 87)

Bow Pose: Dhanurasana

Lie face down, hands by your sides, palms facing up, legs together. Turn your forehead to the floor; bending at the knees, raise your feet, bringing your heels as close to your buttocks as possible. Raise your head, keeping your chin on the floor, then reach back with your hands and grasp your ankles firmly. Pull your hands and legs together to raise your head, chest, knees and thighs off the floor. Raise your entire body weight on your navel. Breathe in and slowly exhale. Hold for 5-10 breaths, then release. Repeat 2-4 times.

Thunderbolt Pose: Vajrasana (see p. 87)

Fish Pose: Matsyasana

Sit on the floor with your spine straight, legs outstretched, feet together and toes pointed (or if this is too difficult, keep your feet relaxed). Lean back and to the right, slightly shifting your position to place your right elbow on the floor behind you. Then, leaning slightly to the left, place your left elbow behind you, on the floor. Slide your hands under your buttocks, pressing your arms and elbows into the floor. Raise your torso and tilt your head back to arch your neck. Breathe in and slowly exhale. Hold for 5-10 breaths, then release. Repeat 2-4 times.

Spinal Twist Pose I: Vakrasana

Sit on the floor with your legs together and outstretched, hands flat behind you, on the floor. Bring your palms near your buttocks. Bend your right knee and place your right foot to the inside of your left knee. Twist your torso, bringing your left shoulder and hand towards your right knee, and tuck your right knee into your left armpit. Keep your right hand on the floor behind you. Twist your neck and body as far as is comfortable towards your right hand. Breathe in and then slowly exhale. Hold for 5-10 breaths, then slowly release. Repeat on the other side. Repeat the sequence 2-4 times.

Spinal Twist Pose II: Sulabha Matsyendrasana

Sit on the floor, legs outstretched and ankles about 3-4 inches apart. Bend your right knee and bring it straight up to your chest. Bend your left knee so that it points to the left, and keep it near the floor. Use your hands to position your left foot at or near the crotch. Move your right foot to the left side of your body, and use your left hand to place your right ankle behind your left knee. Hook your right big toe with your left index finger and tuck your right knee into your left armpit, or just place your left hand on your knee. Keep your buttocks on the floor. Twist your upper body to the right and put your right hand on the floor. If you can, bring your right hand around to your lower back. Breathe in and then slowly exhale. Hold for 5-10 breaths, then release. Repeat on the other side. Repeat the sequence 2-4 times.

Leg-lift Pose: Viparitakarini

Lie flat on your back, legs together and outstretched and arms along your sides, palms down. Keeping your knees straight but not locked, contract your abdominal muscles to raise your legs about 6 inches off the floor. If this is too difficult, lie on your back with your buttocks against a wall and your legs raised above you, resting on the wall. Breathe in and then slowly exhale. Hold for 5-10 breaths, then release. Repeat the sequence 2-4 times.

Plough Pose: Halasana (see p. 88)

Downward-facing Dog Pose: Adho Mukha Svanasana

Lie face down, arms bent and palms flat on the floor at the sides of your chest, fingers pointing towards your head. Tuck your toes under and lift up to your hands and knees. Exhaling, press your feet and hands into the floor and raise your buttocks, straightening your knees and pulling your thighs back. Do not lock your knees. Keep your spine straight. Extend your chest back towards your thighs. Keeping your elbows and knees straight but not locked, press your heels into the floor, push your hips up and pull your shoulders down. Breathe in and slowly exhale. Hold for 5-10 breaths, then release. Repeat the entire sequence 2-4 times.

Corpse Pose: Shavasana (see p. 88)

Meditative Breathing: Pranayama

This breathing exercise, called Shitali, produces a cooling effect in the body. Sit comfortably in a cross-legged position and slowly become aware of your breath. Take 10 natural breaths. Partially protrude your tongue and fold up the sides to form a long, narrow tube. Narrow the passage by further pressing the lips around the tongue. Inhale and receive the cold air passing through the tongue tube. Close your mouth and retain the breath for as long as you comfortably can. Exhale through both nostrils. Build up breath-retention time with subsequent practice but only to a level of comfort, and never rush out-breath. 10-15 minutes of pranayama everyday is extremely beneficial for all pitta conditions.

KAPHA YOGA ROUTINE

Kapha imbalances are generally indicated by swelling, congestion and a general feeling of heaviness. The metabolism is slowed down, which leaves you feeling cold and sluggish all the time, and constantly perspiring. Yoga routines that balance kapha focus on stimulating the mind and creating a feeling of lightness in the body.

Stomach Lock: Uddiyana Bandha (see p. 87)

Posterior Stretch Pose: Pashchimottasana

Sit on the floor, legs outstretched, arms alongside your body. Bending your trunk slowly, try to hook your fingers around your big toes (or grasp your calves or ankles if you are less flexible). Slowly, bend farther forward, stretching your trunk along your thighs, and rest your face on your knees. Breathe in and then slowly exhale. Hold for 5-10 breaths, then release. Repeat 2-4 times.

Seated Mountain Pose: Parvatasana

Sit on the floor, legs outstretched and spread as wide as is comfortable. Bend your right knee, and place your heel at the crotch. Bend your left leg and place your left foot under your right leg. Keep your spine straight. Flatten your palms together at your diaphragm, just below the middle of your chest and above your abdominal muscles, projecting your elbows outward. Raise your joined palms along the centre line of your body to the level of the lips, then nose, then forehead, then above the head, lengthening towards the sky. Your upper arms should touch your ears. Experience the pull from hips to fingertips. Breathe in and then slowly exhale. Hold for 5-10 breaths, then release. Repeat 2-4 times.

Spinal Twist Pose I: Vakrasana (see p. 91)

Cat Pose: Maharjasana

Sit on your heels with your knees hip-width apart and toes on the floor. Position your palms on the floor in front of you at shoulder-width distance and lean forward, bringing your hips up over your knees. Inhale, relax your trunk and stretch your head and neck backward, curving your spine and pressing towards the floor as far as is comfortable. Close your eyes and relax your stomach. Exhale, lower your head and neck and raise your back up, this time arching your spine as far as is comfortable. Release, relax your neck and hang your head down, drawing your chin to your chest. Repeat 5-10 times.

Tall Tree Pose: Tadasana

Stand with your feet hip-width apart, hands at your sides. Raise your arms in front of you to shoulder height, palms facing down. Continue to raise your hands over your head while also raising your heels slowly. Stretch your arms fully, with your upper arms hugging your ears and your palms facing each other. Keep your heels together and balance. Breathe in and then slowly exhale. Hold or 5-10 breaths, then slowly release. Repeat 2-4 times.

Adapted Wheel Pose: Parivartachakrasana

Stand with your feet hip-width apart, hands at your sides. Slowly, raise both arms sideways to shoulder height. Bend towards your left side, still facing front. Drop your left arm to rest along your left thigh. Stretch your right arm above your shoulder, keeping it near your right ear, and slowly bend at the waist to your left, taking care not to strain yourself. With your right foot firmly on the floor, stretch upward towards your right fingertips. Breathe in and then slowly exhale. Hold for 5-10 breaths, then slowly release. Repeat on the other side. Repeat the sequence 2-4 times.

Camel Pose: Ustrasana

Kneel with the tops of your feet on the floor and your body straight and tall. Exhale and press your pelvis forward, leaning back gradually and lifting your chest. Reach back to your feet and grasp your heels, or just rest your hands on the back of your pelvis. Lean your head back, keeping your thighs perpendicular to the floor. Breathe in and then slowly exhale. Hold for 5-10 breaths, then slowly release. Repeat 2-4 times.

Boat Pose: Naukasana/Navasana

Lie face down, chin to one side and hands at your sides. Turn your forehead to the floor, bring your palms to chest level then stretch your arms ahead of you, palms down. Contracting the muscles of the buttocks, waist, back and neck, raise your upper body from abdomen to fingertips while raising your lower body from abdomen to toes. Raise all parts high, keeping your elbows and knees straight but not locked. Breathe in and then slowly exhale. Hold for 5-10 breaths, then slowly release. Repeat 2-4 times.

Metabolic Asana Series

This series of poses is designed to raise your heart rate and create the heat that kaphas need. Stand with your feet 3-4 feet apart, arms lifted to your sides at shoulder height and toes turned out. Bend your arms and point your hands up to the sky. Exhale and squat, then inhale and straighten to stand. Keep your back straight and abdomen tight. Repeat this 10 times. Jump with your feet together and squat all the way down to the floor. Keeping your palms strong on the floor, exhale and jump with your feet backward, straightening your legs and raising your buttocks into the downward-facing dog position (p. 92). Then inhale and jump with your feet forward, returning to the squat position with your feet between your hands. Exhale and jump with your feet back one more time into the downward-facing dog position. Jump with your feet together or walk your hands back to your feet. Repeat the squat and downward-facing dog series 10 times. Straighten your legs and slowly stand upright. Repeat the entire sequence 3-7 times.

Meditative Breathing: Pranayama

This breathing exercise, called Kapalbhati, cleanses the nasal passages in the head and improves the functioning of the diaphragm. Sit back on your heels, hands resting loosely on your knees, and slowly become aware of your breath. Take 10 natural breaths. Open your mouth very slightly. Expand your abdomen while inhaling and contract your abdomen while exhaling. Quickly alternate inhalation and exhalation, with accompanying expansion and contraction of the abdomen, to strongly activate your abdominal muscles for 30 breaths. This completes 1 round. Rest and repeat for 30 breaths. 2-5 rounds of this pranayama performed everyday is extremely beneficial for addressing kapha imbalances.

FIVE

Eating for Balance

We all know that eating properly is crucial to good health. With the principles of Ayurveda, you can go even further in understanding how attention to diet can improve your quality of life. According to Ayurveda, everything about your eating habits has a strong effect on the mind and body; not only which foods and herbs you eat but also the amount you eat, the timing of your meals and snacks and the combinations of flavours all influence your wellbeing. The food you eat can have medicinal and therapeutic effects beyond mere sustenance. When you eat well, in every sense, you maximize your vitality (ojas). Ayurveda recommends whole, nutritious foods and eating patterns that are tailored to balance your dosha type.

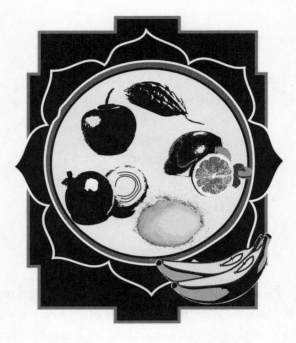

Poor digestion, stemming from an unbalanced diet, is one of the first signs of ill health. When your digestive energies, known as agni (digestive fire) are robust, you create healthy tissues, eliminate waste products efficiently and maximize ojas. On the other hand, if your agni is weakened, digestion is incomplete and creates ama or toxins that get stored in the body.

Indigestion disturbs the doshas at their core, in the gastrointestinal tract. When your diet is off-balance, not only are food nutrients not easily absorbed but they can also accumulate as toxins. People feel the effects of poor digestion differently: kapha dosha imbalances originate in the upper digestive tract (i.e., the stomach); pitta imbalances prey on the mid-digestive tract (i.e., the small intestine); and vata imbalances are felt in the lower digestive tract (i.e., the colon).

There is no 'Ayurveda diet' and there are no 'bad' foods in Ayurveda – there is only the idea of balance. A harmonious diet balances not only nutritional qualities, but also taste and even the heating or cooling energetic effects a food has on you after it is digested. (Heating foods are those that are stimulating, such as black pepper; cooling foods are those that are sedating or can produce sluggishness, such as bread. Sattwic foods, such as almonds, create mental clarity and balance.) It takes into account individual items such as fruit, meats and vegetables as well as the meals that they combine into once cooked. While there is an emphasis on fruit and vegetables, and many Indians are vegetarian, Ayurveda in itself does not prescribe vegetarianism. In fact, a whole array of meats and fish are emphasized in the ancient texts. But Ayurvedic doctors do recommend a pure and close-to-nature (sattwic) diet with plenty of fresh fruit, vegetables, nuts and seeds combined with herbs and spices to purify and balance the mind and body.

THE 6 TASTES (RASAS)

Understanding the concept of rasa is critical for under-standing the nutritional as well as the medicinal value of foods. In Ayurveda, there are 6 different tastes, each of which has a post-digestive effect on the doshas that influence the way we feel and how much energy we have. Most foods are a combination of more than one taste. Influenced by Western nutritional practices, today we think of a balanced meal as one which combines fibre, carbohydrates, proteins and fats, but in Ayurveda, a balanced meal is one that combines all 6 tastes. We can tailor each meal to dosha-specific needs by having more of some tastes than others. We can then further customize the diet for corrective benefits. A healthy person is able to enjoy all of the 6 tastes, but if we have an imbalance, or vikruti, we sometimes develop an aversion to foods with similar qualities as the doshas that are imbalanced. These foods are then no longer palatable, no longer medicinal and can even become bad for us. For example, if you have too much pitta, then spicy foods and chilli may not appeal to you. To restore balance, a change of diet is key. The positive and negative influences of each taste are detailed below.

SWEET

Foods with a sweet taste are calming and soothing to the system. Their grounding qualities balance vata and their cooling qualities balance pitta. But taken in excess, these foods can imbalance kapha, creating heaviness and slowing digestion. Sweet foods include not just sugar- and honey-based foods but also butter, milk, sesame seeds, fruit and vegetables with a naturally sweet taste (such as banana or sweet potato, and carbohydrates such as oats, rice or wheat bread.

SALTY

Foods with a salty taste enhance digestion. Their warming qualities balance vata but, taken in excess, they can disturb kapha and pitta, leading to water retention and inflammation. Salty foods include dried or salted pickles and snack foods, any soy or salted chilli sauce.

SOUR

Foods with a sour taste stimulate digestion. Their warming qualities balance vata but, taken in excess, they will disturb kapha and pitta, increasing body weight and skin sensitivity. Some examples are yogurt and buttermilk, pineapple, raw tomato, lemon and fermented foods such as vinegar, chilli and pickles.

PUNGENT

Foods with a pungent taste decongest the body, increasing digestion. Their drying and heating properties balance kapha but, taken in excess, these foods can disturb pitta and vata by creating excess heat and dryness inside the body. Pungent foods include mustard, raw onion and pickles, and hot spices like chilli, peppers, caraway seeds and black pepper.

BITTER

Foods with a bitter taste create lightness and clarity. They balance kapha and pitta but, taken in excess, they aggravate vata, including dryness in the skin. Examples of bitter foods are karela (bitter melon), aloe vera and dark, leafy green vegetables like spinach and mustard greens.

ASTRINGENT

Foods with an astringent taste create lightness. Their cooling properties balance pitta and their drawing properties balance kapha but, taken in excess, these foods can disturb vata, leading to dryness and flatulence. Examples of astringent foods are pomegranate, cabbage, lemon, apple and chickpea.

For a meal to be balanced, it is important that we pay attention to the order in which we experience the 6 tastes. These are digested in a specific order based on doshas. Sweet and salty tastes both are digested in the stomach, the first part of the gastrointestinal tract, by the kapha dosha. Therefore, these foods should be eaten first. Sour tastes are digested in the small intestine by the pitta dosha. They should be eaten next. Pungent, bitter and astringent tastes are digested in the colon by the vata dosha and should be eaten last.

Unlike Western meals which are typically served in courses, in India small portions of food representing each of the 6 tastes are assembled together on large platters called thalis. This way, diners can pick and choose what food to eat in the preferred order and also adjust the intake of the tastes according to the doshas they are aiming to balance.

TIPS FOR PERFECT DIGESTION

Your constitution, or dosha, is affected by not just your food intake, but also by how you eat – how you feel when you eat and how long you take to have a meal, even when you snack. Follow the simple principles below to ensure optimal digestion.

- Maintain a state of calm while eating. Eating under stressful circumstances turns your body into a pressure cooker, causing fermentation of the food in your digestive tract. This causes toxins to be absorbed into the bloodstream and even creates gas. Stress includes anything that takes away enjoyment from eating – from watching violent TV shows to discussing difficult situations.
- Condition yourself to drinking water that is slightly warm or at room temperature, rather than ice-cold water, as this dampens agni, or the 'digestive fire',

responsible for digesting food efficiently for maximum ojas. Avoid water right before your meal; it is better to have water between meals. If possible, have 2 glasses of warm water upon rising and a glass of warm water or herbal tea following meals.

- Chew your food completely, without rushing. Foods that are not completely chewed and broken down in the mouth make for harder work for the stomach. This often leads to pain and discomfort during or right after your meal.

- Make lunch the largest meal of the day. Digestive power is strongest when the sun shines directly overhead, so lunch should be your main meal, as the food has the best chance of being most efficiently digested. This is also the best meal to involve more complex food. In the mornings and evenings, the system tends to be more sluggish. Therefore, breakfast and dinner should be smaller and comprised of easily digestible foods, such as fruit for breakfast and lightly cooked vegetables, stews and soups for dinner.

- Eat nutritious, whole foods. Canned or over-processed foods that have lost their colour and flavour will have also lost their nutritional value. Also be careful how much you cook your fresh foods, especially vegetables. Indian chefs will tell you that when it comes to food, what you see is what you get – the more the colours in your thali, the more nutritious your meal. Select foods that are whole and organic. These have raw vitality and can best balance your doshas in the way that nature intended them to.

- Adjust food quantities according to your dosha. Vata types have a smaller food-intake capacity but a more rapid metabolism. They often need 4-5 smaller meals in a day to give them the vital energy that keeps them functioning optimally. Pitta types have a strong metabolism and do well with 3 regular meals a day. Kapha types have slow metabolism, and should eat 2-3 meals a day and avoid snacking.

- Do not eat until after you have digested your previous meal. Eating too soon after your last meal causes bloating, acidity and gas. While we all have different rates of digestion, rule of thumb tells us that we have completely digested a meal when we feel a sensation of lightness both physically and emotionally. This could be anywhere from 2-4 hours after a meal, but be sure to think about how you feel rather than look at the clock.

- Eat sensible portions. It is easy to be lured by the appeal of gourmet foods and eat more than is appropriate. Starving yourself to follow a trendy diet is just as bad. At each meal, the volume of your food should equal 1 anjali, or about 2 handfuls. This fills most of the stomach, the rest being left empty to allow food to mix freely with the digestive juices and vata energy to push it down through the digestive tract. Fasting is not prescribed in Ayurveda – it weakens ojas, compromising strength and complexion.

- Follow your meal with digestive munchies or mukhwas. These are eaten at the end of a meal to help encourage digestion. Eating a teaspoon of mukhwas is a great after-meal ritual. Make your own from equal parts sesame seeds, whole cumin seeds and fennel seeds, and keep the mix in a jar in a cool, dry place.

EATING FOR YOUR DOSHA

Once you have identified your dosha, experiment with making a few changes to your diet that will help keep your body in balance. Of course, you will not be able to stick to these guidelines all the time, but being conscious of your body's natural tendencies is a great way to help control your moods, keep your energy up and maximize your ojas.

VATA

- Eat many small meals throughout the day to help sustain your energy level.
- Eat warm, cooked, light foods with sweet, salty and sour tastes. Avoid cold foods like ice cream and chilled purées.
- Moisten dry or raw foods, bread and omelette with ghee (see p. 33), oil or butter.
- Avoid caffeine in excess.

- Substitute brown sugar, honey or maple syrup for white sugar.
- Avoid gassy, bloating foods such as dry dals, beans and soft drinks. If you really enjoy dals and beans, cook them with ghee and digestion-aiding spices such as ginger, cardamom, cinnamon, coriander and dill.
- Favour root vegetables and leafy greens for your vegetable consumption. Do not, however, eat them raw; cook them, preferably with pure ghee or sesame oil.
- Eat plenty of yogurt in the warmer months and drink a cup of warm milk daily in the cooler months.
- Eat fleshy fruit such as peach, mango and papaya. Drink plenty of citrus fruit and vegetable juices. Amla juice is an excellent choice.
- Do not mix different types of animal protein such as fish and eggs, milk and meat, or chicken and shellfish.
- Avoid low-fat diets. Vata types need the nutritious quality of fats.
- Sip a specially blended vata tea (available at speciality stores) to help regularize digestion in the colon, or try salty lassi.

PITTA

- Eat 3 meals a day with lunch as your main meal.
- Eat cooling and light foods with sweet and bitter tastes.

- Avoid caffeine, alcohol, salt or spices in excess.
- Substitute brown sugar for honey, maple syrup or white sugar.
- Avoid yeast-risen breads. Choose roti and rice with ghee (see p. 33) and sprinkled with cooling digestive herbs such as coriander, parsley and dill.
- Favour leafy greens for your vegetable consumption. Bitter greens are your best bet and are plentiful through the year. Vary your selection, choosing from spinach, mustard, kale and collard greens.
- Eat plenty of sweet fruit such as sweet cherry, red grapes or fig. Avoid sour citrus fruit and juices, such as grapefruit. Drink plenty of green drinks such as parsley, celery, fresh neem or wheatgrass juice. An excellent drink for pitta is equal parts vegetable juice and coconut milk, enhanced with a teaspoon of either aloe vera or spirulina.
- Avoid foods such as mustard, hard yellow cheeses, red meat, tomato and eggplant. These heating foods further incense the fiery pitta qualities.
- Sip a specially blended pitta tea (available in speciality stores) to balance acidity and soothe your stomach, or drink milk or cranberry juice.

KAPHA

- Make sure that dinner is the lightest meal of the day and try to eat no later than sunset. Soups and light vegetable stews make ideal dinners.

- Eat warm, dry, light foods with bitter, pungent and astringent tastes.
- Avoid heavy oils and butter or fried, fatty foods. Opt for lighter oils such as olive or canola oil.
- Avoid caffeine and sugar in excess.
- Avoid heavy, congestive foods that are difficult to digest such as pastas, breads and cakes.
- Eat plenty of dark leafy green and brightly coloured vegetables like celery, carrot, spinach and tomato.
- Eat plenty of citrus fruit and berries. Drink citrus fruit and vegetable juices.
- Avoid having more than 3 meals in a day and maintain a gap of at least 4 hours between meals. Also, avoid snacking between meals.
- Avoid high-protein diets for extended periods.
- Sip a specially blended kapha tea (available in speciality stores) to balance digestion in the stomach and prevent discomfort during and after mealtimes. Also try salty lassi (an Indian beverage made from yogurt and water), buttermilk or lemonade.
- Flush your system with water throughout the day.

SIX

Ritucharya

Seasons of Ayurveda

While you practise Ayurvedic dinacharya year-round, it is important that you try to match your lifestyle rhythm to that of the season and the geography around you. Just like a person, the environment and seasons are characterized by the 3 doshas, each of which is more active and influential at different times of the year.

The change in Ayurvedic seasons affects the balance of the doshas. While any one dosha might dominate your constitution, remember that you are made of all 3, and that these might be thrown off-balance by the strong influence of the dosha of the season. If you do not shift your nutritional and lifestyle patterns to balance what is

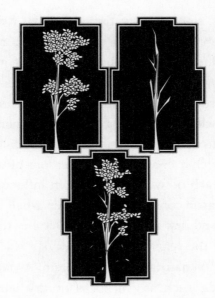

happening in the environment, the dosha within you that is the same as the dosha of the season will be thrown off course. This does not mean that you have to completely reinvent your life several times a year, but merely that you should make small changes to live in harmony with the seasons. While the supermarket can provide all foods all year round, it is wise to eat warming foods in winter and cooling fruits in summer. Try eating fresh produce, fruit and vegetables that are available through farms and suppliers close to where you live to be sure that you are in tune with the season. You might also want to change your yoga routine – the secret here lies in your ability to adjust and adapt accordingly to the needs of the season's dosha. Also, since each of the doshas has a tendency to become aggravated during the season prior to that of its peak influence, it is ideal at the onset of its season of influence. Ayurveda suggests 3 such detox retreats or cleansing programmes during the year – at the onset of the season where each dosha is at peak influence.

The Ayurvedic year can be roughly divided into 3 seasons (which overlap with the 4 seasons of the Western calendar), each of which has its own influencing dosha. The vata season consists of the winter, when the weather turns cold and dry, approximately October to March. At this time of the year you can eat heavier, warming foods with plenty of natural oils and protein. Avoid salads and drying foods, such as chickpeas or dry lentils, during this season, as these will exacerbate vata. Winter meals prepared with nourishing foods such as nuts, meats and warm and creamy soups, stews or casseroles are ideal for the vata season. Exercising indoors is preferable at this time of the year to avoid the onslaught of wind and cold temperatures which can further exacerbate vata. You tend to feel more tired at this time of the year, so slow down and make things easy on yourself. It is ideal to conduct a vata detox retreat in October, right at the onset of the vata season.

The kapha season runs from late winter to spring, approximately March to June. Flowers begin to bud during this cool, damp time of the year. Eat light, fresh foods such as vegetable soups and light stews during this season. Avoid dairy foods, ice cream and excess oils as they naturally aggravate kapha. In many cultures, this is the time of the year for spring festivals, which wake people into action after the sleepy wintertime. It is a good idea to lead an all-round more active lifestyle now, whether this means taking brisk walks or keeping yourself mentally and physically occupied with reading or aerobic activity; avoid napping. This is the season of undertaking projects. Kapha detox retreats conducted in late January or February, before the onset of the kapha season, will help you combat congestion, allergies and sluggishness during this time of the year.

The pitta season runs from summer into early autumn, approximately June to October. This is the time when the sun is strongest overhead and the fire element is at peak influence. To compensate, eat colder, sweeter foods and cool drinks. Avoid hot, spicy foods and excess alcohol, as these create inflammation. Choose moderate exercise that tones the muscles without causing you to overheat, such as walking and swimming. During these months, avoid inverted postures, such as head stands, in your yoga practice. And remember, the days are long now, so get plenty of rest and, if possible, take short naps. This will help you stay calm and collected in many situations. As with the other seasons, it is ideal to undergo a pitta detox retreat in April or May, before you are into the thick of the season.

SEASONAL DETOX RETREAT

A detoxification programme is ideal for eliminating dosha imbalances that naturally build up through the seasons. The classic Ayurvedic detoxification is called panchakarma, an intensive programme of invasive therapies that require the supervision of a physician. While panchakarma is beneficial, it is not easily available nor essential for maintaining strong ojas, unless your doshas are severely out of balance and are causing illness. Checking into an Ayurvedic spa to undergo a short detox programme based on purvakarma, the nutritional and body therapies that support panchakarma, 3 times a year is ideal, as the staff will be able to guide you with treatments, food, yoga and other activities that will help restore balance and maximum vitality. However, given the time and expense, it is good to know how to follow your own simple detox programme at home. The programme described here is a simple 3-day one that can be easily done at home over a weekend. The key to a successful detox is to stay focused and shut out the rest of the world, allowing you both emotional and physical release. The detox guidelines below are ideal for any dosha season, or can be customized with foods and herbs for the season at hand. Remember to use your judgment – detoxifying is not advised for children, pregnant or nursing mothers, or people who have been diagnosed with an illness or are taking strong medication.

THE WEEK BEFORE

To prepare for your detox, it is important to loosen and liquefy toxins and bring them to the superficial tissue layers. For 7 days before your retreat, follow your normal personal-care routine, but start each day by drinking a ¼ to ½ cup of warmed ghee (see p. 33). Follow this with an astringent liquid like orange juice or hot water with fresh lemon juice to help take away the aftertaste (this will also help encourage bowel elimination). Try to get into the habit of emptying your bowels soon after consuming this drink. In addition, drink 8-10 cups of warm water through the day.

FRIDAY

Begin the detox retreat with a cleansing ritual. Start your day with ghee and hot lemon water as per the previous 7 days. Then, using a tongue scraper or just a toothbrush, scrape your tongue from back to front 6-7 times, followed by your normal personal-care routine. Eat as lightly as possible through the day: try to avoid heavy proteins, carbohydrates, sweets and fried foods. Also avoid soda, coffee and tea. As with the previous 7 days, drink 8-10 cups of warm water through the day.

Evening Meal

When you come home from work, eat a light meal, such as a seasonal vegetable salad and a bowl of vegetable soup. On the side, have some toasted rye bread without butter. Drink a cup of triphala tea following your meal: boil 1 teaspoon of triphala herbs (see p. 35) in 4 ounces of hot water. This gentle laxative will help remove toxins throughout the digestive system. Be sure not to sweeten the tea. Have dinner by 6 pm, so that you will have plenty of time to sip herbal tea through the remainder of the evening. Vatas should replace the salad with a fistful of cooked seasonal vegetables dressed with plenty of sesame oil and fresh herbs and seasoning; they may spread ghee (see p. 33) on the rye toast. Pittas should make sure that their vegetable soup has an even mixture of green and coloured seasonal vegetables.

Face and Neck Massage

Giving yourself a 20-minute face and neck massage with a dosha facial oil will help ease headaches and relieve tension and anxiety (see pp. 46-47). Throughout the massage, focus on releasing tension in your neck by letting go of your head and allowing it to become heavier and heavier, creating pressure against your hands.

Meditative Breathing (Pranayama)

In a well-ventilated room, sit comfortably in a cross-legged position on the floor or in a straight-backed chair. Close your eyes and relax your body. Try to shut out distractions from your mind so that you can completely focus on your breath. If your mind wanders, observe the thought, let it pass then bring your attention back to your breath. As you become aware of your breath, breathe in for a count of 3, hold briefly then breathe out for a count of 6. If you are able to do so, increase the length of your in-breath and out-breath, but make sure that you always maintain the 1:2 proportion with a brief hold between each complete round. Continue several rounds this way – at least 50 rounds or 5 minutes, whichever comes first. Next, breathe normally for another 5 minutes or so, focusing on your breath without counting. Finally, focus on the part of your nose where the coolness of your in-breath meets the warmth of your out-breath. Remain focused on this and then think of a positive emotion. Nurture it and resolve to further it. Remain focused on this emotion for a few minutes before you gradually come out of your meditation.

Ending Your Day

Avoid television or loud music today. Try to avoid reading, as it is important that you focus inward and clear yourself of thoughts and stimuli. Go to sleep early, as you will need to wake up early on Saturday. Prepare a copper vessel with an infusion of herbs in warm water and leave to stand overnight (see pp. 34-36 for herbs).

SATURDAY AND SUNDAY

Throughout these 2 days, drink water and herbal teas; aim to drink 10-12 glasses of water and as much herbal tea as you would like. Be sure to drink warm, not iced, water: iced water dampens the digestive fire (agni) that is responsible for efficient digestion.

Waking Up

On both these days, wake up slowly, joyously remembering that the day is dedicated to you. Make yourself a hot lemon drink by squeezing the juice of half a lemon into 1 cup of herb-infused water from the copper vessel you prepared the night before. Heat the water and sip it slowly to begin your body's natural detox processes. Go to the bathroom and try to empty your bowels, but remember not to strain or push yourself.

Nasal Cleansing and Tongue Scraping

Splash your face and eyes with cold water. Then, using a neti pot, cleanse both nostrils with 1 tablespoon mustard oil mixed into 1 pot of dosha herbal tea and a pinch of salt (see pp. 82-83 for complete instructions). Use at least 2 pots per nostril. Using a tongue scraper or toothbrush, scrape your tongue from back to front at 6-7 times to get rid of toxins.

Skin – Brushing and Self-massage (Abhyanga)

Give yourself an invigorating dry skin brushing with a rough towel or natural loofah to help slough off the dead skin cells that can clog your pores, helping your skin to breathe better. Skin brushing stimulates the lymphatic system and helps revitalize the skin. Brush all over, starting with your arms and legs and working inward towards the heart. Applying only as much pressure as is comfortable, brush until your skin becomes warm, but do not overdo it as it can cause your skin to redden excessively: 5 minutes or so is plenty. Follow the brushing with an abhyanga massage (see p. 43) and feel the oils penetrate into the pores. Pitta types might be a little more sensitive, and you should be careful not to brush on broken or irritated skin.

Morning Yoga

Start Saturday and Sunday with a rejuvenating yoga practice. Follow the appropriate yoga routine for the dosha of the season, as outlined in Chapter 4. End with alternate nostril breathing, a yogic technique that harmonizes your energy and strengthens respiration.

In this pranayama, the out-breath is twice as long as the in-breath and so efficiently clears waste products from lungs and body. Do not strain your breath, but focus on keeping it long, steady and deep, building rhythm and intensity as you go along.

Close your right nostril with your right thumb and exhale completely through your left nostril. Inhale through your left nostril to a count of 4. Close your left nostril with your ring finger and little finger, holding your index and middle fingers to the bridge of your nose. Hold for a count of 4. (If you can, build this up to a count of 8.) Release your right nostril, exhaling completely for a count of 8. Close the right nostril and keep both nostrils closed for a count of 4 (or 8 if you can). Repeat the sequence on the other side. This sequence is 1 round. Repeat the breathing technique for at least 15 rounds, or better still, for 10-15 minutes.

Breakfast

For the first meal on each of these 2 days, eat a large bowl of fruit salad with a tall glass of freshly squeezed orange juice or dosha herbal tea. This meal will help the liver begin ridding the body of accumulated waste matter. Vata types benefit from adding a handful of sesame, sunflower or pumpkin seeds for constitutional warmth. Pitta types might find orange juice too acidic, and may substitute it with pitta tea or any other fresh fruit juice of the season. You may also prepare a blended fruit smoothie in place of the salad: in a blender, combine a large banana with half a cup of your choice of seasonal fresh fruit, a spoonful of chyawanprash and half a cup of water to thin it out.

DETOX SPA TREATMENTS

If you are visiting an Ayurvedic centre for detoxifying, take advantage of the available face and body treatments while you are there, as they help loosen and expel toxins. If you are detoxifying at home, undertaking these treatments will aid the rejuvenation experience. Follow the suggestions below for a comprehensive Ayurvedic home-spa experience.

SATURDAY

Face and body scrub with ubtan: Prepare a cleansing ubtan scrub (see p. 56). Work the scrub all over your face and body to improve circulation and tone slack muscles. Rinse with warm water.

Herbal steam: This is a great practice to eliminate toxins. Steam your face over a bowl of hot water combined with 2 handfuls of seasonal herbs (see pp. 34-36) for about 10 minutes. Hold your face at least 12 inches above the water and tent your head and the bowl with a towel to prevent the steam from escaping. (Vata types, who may find steam alone to be too drying, can apply a little sesame oil to the face and neck before steaming.) Pat your face dry and splash with tepid water to refresh the skin. Run a hot shower to generate steam and rest in the steam 7-10 minutes to purify the skin of the body as well.

Lepa Mask: This mask absorbs impurities from the skin. Mix together a mask (see pp. 63-67) and apply it all over the face and body. Leave it on for about 15 minutes and try to remain as still as possible. (Vata types may add a few tablespoons of sesame oil to the mixture if they find it too drying.) Rinse with water.

Rinse: Rinse your face and body with a mixture of 1 tablespoon cider vinegar diluted in 4 ounces of water. The cider vinegar is an excellent natural toner.

Moisturize: Massage your face and body with aloe vera gel for pittas or heavy whipped cream for vatas and kaphas to soften and refresh your skin.

SUNDAY

On Saturday, you cared for your skin; on Sunday, focus on your hair, hands and feet.

Hair and Scalp: Cleanse and oil the hair (see pp. 71-73). This will help condition, detoxify and supply nutrients to your hair and scalp. Leave the oil in for as long as possible. Rinse thoroughly, then apply a nourishing protein mask to your scalp made from ½ cup yogurt, 1 tablespoon lemon juice, 1 egg and 2 tablespoons brahmi powder (if available; see p. 34). Leave this mask on for about 20 minutes, then rinse thoroughly.

Hands and Feet: With a loofah or rough hand towel, gently massage your hands and feet to increase circulation. Then soak your hands and feet in a tub of warm water infused with any of your favourite essential oils. Use a pumice stone to ease out any rough areas on the feet. Warm 3-4 tablespoons of ghee (see p. 33) and rub generously into your hands and feet, massaging as per the instructions outlined in Chapter 3. This will moisturize, relieve tension and prevent water retention. If you have cold extremities, keep your hands and feet warm for a resting period by wrapping them in a hot, wet towel that has been wrung dry and wrapped in another dry towel.

DOWNTIME

During your detox programme, spend part of the morning as you like – reading an interesting book, listening to music, writing in your journal, gardening, painting – do whatever you enjoy. It is important to spend time unwinding and doing what you want to rather than what you think you should do.

LUNCH

After your morning yoga and spa therapies, enjoy a large raw salad made with fresh vegetables of the season (vata types should have a cooked vegetable salad). Choose from the dosha-balancing herbs and spices listed in Chapter 5 and Ayurvedic Pantry (see pp. 32-37) to add flavour. Eat your lunch slowly and mindfully, focusing on the flavours and textures of the ingredients. While you eat, reflect on the view from your window, or even the sight of indoor plants and flowers, to unlock the mind.

REST

Rest is important to calm the mind and allow the physical body to deal with fatigue as it detoxifies. After lunch take some quiet time to listen to music, read or take a short nap for half an hour to an hour if you are sleepy. If you are tired but cannot fall asleep, simply rest your mind and body by lying down and emptying your mind of thoughts.

EXERCISE

Your detox retreat will be enhanced by a brisk walk, preferably in the open air so that you can breathe in natural oxygen directly into your lungs (during the chill of the vata season or in northern climates, you may use a treadmill). Staying aware of good posture, warm up by starting out slow and then build to a brisk pace. Keep your chest out, swing your arms wide and breathe through your mouth. Walk for 20-30 minutes, with the goal being 1 hour. If you prefer other types of exercise, consult the chart on pp. 130-32 for modes of exercise appropriate to the dosha of the relevant season.

MUSICAL MEDITATION

When you begin to feel the effects of your detox, musical meditation is ideal. Put on some of your favourite music. Try to choose music that evokes the positive emotions for the dosha of the season (see pp. 112-15). To do this, select music that reminds you of the emotion you are focusing on. For example, during a vata seasonal detox programme, choose music that is calming and provides focus. Mantras are ideal. During a pitta seasonal detox programme, choose music that reinforces love and respect for the people you know. The music can be of any genre – jazz, classical, easy listening, Vedic chanting, instrumental – but avoid loud, jarring, disturbing sounds or controversial music of any kind. Spend at least half an hour listening to the music and thinking about a time or situation in your life when you most felt the emotion evoked by it. This could be when you were young, or it could be recently. Try to take yourself deeper into this emotion and plan how you can carry it through to new experiences in your life. Feel your state of mind uplifted with this new, positive emotion.

DIGESTIVE MEDITATION AND CARE

This is an ideal time to tune into your digestive system and become familiar with it. Place your hands first on your stomach and become aware of any internal movement, feelings or sounds. Do the same with your small intestine in the midriff area and then with the area under your navel or colon. Mentally prepare for your next meal by noticing whether you are hungry or not. Resolve to eat only as much as you need to fill three-quarters of your stomach (this typically translates to about as much food as will fit into both your cupped hands). Using a little oil, massage your stomach in circles, moving clockwise. This will help ease digestion of the last meal and prepare for the next.

DINNER

Dinner during detox should consist of steamed vegetables. Use fresh, green seasonal vegetables, the greener the better. For extra flavour, add fresh herbs such as rosemary, basil, parsley and sage, or pine nuts, sesame seeds and pumpkin seeds. Vata types may add a bit of oil to their vegetables. As with lunch, eat slowly and mindfully, allowing for complete digestion. An hour or so after dinner, follow with triphala tea (see p. 118).

AMUSEMENTS

This is your time to spend doing things that are creative and mindful, yet relaxing. These can be anything from light reading to working the Sunday crossword to needlework or organizing photographs. Do something you enjoy and perhaps do not often get a chance to do during your regular weekly schedule. Think about why you enjoy the activity and the kind of satisfaction or creative stimulus you derive from it. Be thankful for this time to pursue it.

AFTER THE WEEKEND

As you come out of your detox programme, do not return immediately to your regular eating habits. Eat light foods such as vegetable soup, khichdi or a light rice-and-mung-dal dish. Avoid heavy foods like meat, dairy and bread for at least a day or two, as they will be hard to digest right after your detox retreat.

Coming out of the detox retreat, you will more than likely feel tired, perhaps a little heavy-headed and somewhat 'out of it'. Your moods and emotions may be heightened, so you might feel extra weepy, chatty, quiet or low. It is important to recognize these as signs of active detoxifying and not worry about them as unusual or associated with feeling ill. As with your diet, it is important that you gradually readjust to normal life and do not rush back into a frenzied pace.

DOSHA SEASONAL DETOX GUIDELINES

Each season's detox calls for particular elements, whether specific thoughts to meditate on or specific herbs to use cleansing and massage. This chart will help you determine which dosha dominates the season you are experiencing and the appropriate remedies to balance your prakruti in that season. For more information about facial, massage and body therapies, see Chapter 7.

Vata Season (Autumn to Winter)	
Modes of exercise	Yoga, Tai Chi, dance
Positive emotions for meditation	Focus, calm
Herbal teas	Vata tea, ginger tea, brahmi tea, ashwagandha tea
Facial and body abhyanga (massage) oil	Vata oils
Herb-infused water for copper vessel	Ginger and fennel
Facial massage and body therapies	Day 1: Abhyanga, Lepa, Nadi Sveda
	Day 2: Tan Lepa, Pizichil, Shirodhara
Aromatherapy oils	Sandalwood, jatamansi, rose, mandarin
Herbs for facial steaming	Ginger and mixed herbs
Moisturizers	Cream

Pitta Season (Summer to Early Autumn)	
Modes of exercise	Swimming, skiing, basketball
Positive emotions for meditation	Love, respect for others
Herbal teas	Pitta tea, peppermint tea, shatavari tea
Facial and body abhyanga (massage) oil	Pitta oils
Herb-infused water for copper vessel	Coriander
Facial, massage and body therapies	Day 1: Abhyanga, Shirodhara, Svedana
	Day 2: Lepa, Shiro abhyanga, Taila Seka
Aromatherapy oils	Sandalwood, rose, neem, jasmine, tea tree oil, neroli, bitter orange, cinnamon, eucalyptus, black pepper
Herbs for facial steaming	Coriander, basil
Moisturizers	Aloe vera gel (kumari)

Kapha Season (Later Winter to Spring)	
Modes of exercise	Aerobics, cycling, rowing
Positive emotions for meditation	Organizing, creative stimulation
Herbal teas	Kapha tea, ginger-and-lemon tea, triphala tea
Facial and body abhyanga (massage) oil	Kapha oils
Herb-infused water for copper vessel	Ginger and turmeric
Facial, massage and body therapies	Day 1: Abhyanga, Svedana
	Day 2: Udvartana, Shiro abhyanga
Aromatheraphy oils	Cedarwood, juniper, neem
Herbs for facial steaming	Fennel, parsley
Moisturizers	Yogurt

SEVEN

Ayurvedic Body Therapies

Ayurveda tells us that both the physical body and the emotional body can be rejuvenated through massages, facials and body therapies. Some of these treatments call for year-round practice, while others work as seasonal pick-me-ups. While this book is intended as a means to comfortably and easily embrace Ayurvedic practices on your own, a trip to an Ayurvedic spa or wellness centre with expert technicians can provide an excellent education. If you do not live near an Ayurvedic spa, try seeking one out for a yearly or seasonal getaway.

PURVAKARMA

The treatments described in these pages are all part of purvakarma, a series of body therapies performed to

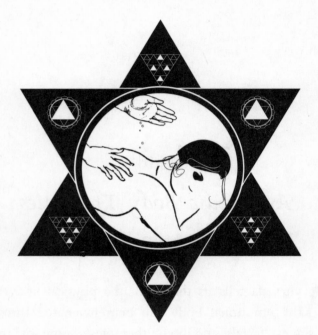

prepare the body to expel toxins through panchakarma or traditional Ayurvedic detox. All purvakarma treatments essentially comprise two procedures:

Snehana (oleation) which makes the body soft and helps loosen toxins

Svedana (fomentation/sweating) which liquefies or melts toxins. Ideally, these can be performed as maintenance on a regular basis but a single session at an Ayurvedic health spa can also be quite effective. Ask the practitioner to focus on your dosha-balancing needs or the dosha-balancing needs of the season, and do not be afraid to ask questions.

SNEHANA THERAPIES

Abhyanga – Massage with Therapeutic Oils

'Abhyanga' literally translates as 'oil application'. Ayurveda provides various oil-massage therapies that relax and detoxify the mind and body. While self-abhyanga benefits you everyday, abhyanga received from a seasoned Ayurvedic technician with appropriate herbal oils prepared from medicinal plants truly meets your body's unique needs. Various styles of abhyanga are available, each distinguished by its own regional Indian flavour. Sometimes the technician will stimulate marma, the vital energy points that awaken immune response. Often, more than one technician will massage your body, rhythmically moving with silent communication like a traditional Indian dance.

Dhara (Oil Therapy)

Dhara means 'flow' – in this case, the flow of therapeutic oils. Of all dhara therapies, Shirodhara is best known for its ability to relieve emotional and physical tension. Warm, herb-infused streaming oil is poured onto the third eye (the area between the eyebrows) and over the forehead to relinquish the negative energies that bring on depression, nervousness, sadness and fatigue. Other dhara therapies include Chakradhara, a treatment in which herbal oils are poured onto the body's subtle energy centres such as the navel, solar plexus and throat to link physical, mental and emotional interactions. In Pizichil or Taila Seka, a rejuvenating herbal oil is simultaneously flowed onto and massaged into the body to rejuvenate the nervous system and relieve inflammation in the joints.

Shiro Abhyanga (Scalp and Spine Massage)

Another critical component of Ayurvedic therapy, this therapy for the central nervous system provides a deep massage of the head, neck and back starting from the base of the spine to release toxic energy upward and out of the crown chakra (energy release point). A completely indulgent experience, it heals through the central chakras and marmas (vital energy points) and helps correct posture. With this physical adjustment, you receive amazing mental clarity and awareness.

SVEDANA THERAPIES

A powerful detoxifying treatment, svedana or sweat therapy helps open the circulatory channels, allowing toxins to be mobilized and eliminated through the sweat glands following abhyanga. A herbal concoction may be added to the steam to further loosen the toxins from the individual. Svedana liquefies the toxins and increases their movement into the gastrointestinal tract.

Svedana can be induced in several ways: through a well-heated chamber (jentaka sveda), medicated steam (nadi sveda), sauna, hot-water bottle, sunbathing, exposure to fire (or use of an infra-red lamp), plasters (anna lepa) and poultices (pinda sveda, bandhana sveda) of hot herbal substances such as mustard, hot baths (avaghana sveda) or showers (especially with medicated oil or water) and hot packs.

After several days (7 or multiples of 7 as prescribed by your Ayurvedic doctor) of abhyanga and svedana, the aggravated doshas become ready to be expelled through the Panchakarma therapy.

OTHER HERBAL BODY THERAPIES

Lepa (Herbal Plaster)

Lepa translates as 'medicinal plaster'. Lepa therapy helps reduce inflammatory swellings and draws out impurities from inside the body to the skin surface. The body is then covered with dosha-specific herbs.

Udvartana (Cleansing)

Udvartana eliminates toxins created by smoking, water retention and environmental poisons. This vigorous massage with fragrant herbal powders stimulates the lymph and cleanses the blood, the skin and the tissues that lie beneath it. Typically, udvartana is combined with a svedana therapy that helps dislodge and release impurities.

Panchakarma

Panchakarma is a Sanskrit word that means '5 actions'. The 5 internally cleansing actions of panchakarma eliminate dosha wastes that have loosened, liquefied and transformed to a physical state by purvakarma therapies.

A highly personalized set of procedures, panchakarma is based on the dosha-balancing needs of the individual. Usually, only parts of the 5 therapies are needed.

Panchakarma therapies fall outside household Ayurveda and are therefore always carried out under the strict supervision of medical personnel. Never try these at home by yourself.

The 5 cleansing actions of panchakarma include:

Vamana

Vamana, an emetic therapy, purifies the body via therapeutic vomiting. It addresses primarily kapha imbalances. Excess kapha toxins that have been brought back to the upper digestive tract (the site of origin for kapha imabalances) through purvakarma therapies are then ejected via emesis.

Virechana

Virechana is a purgative therapy that purifies the body through the lower digestive pathways. It addresses primarily pitta disorders, purifying blood toxins and bile. Excess pitta toxins that have been brought back to the mid-digestive tract (the site of origin for pitta imbalances) are extracted and pushed downward through the colon and out of the body in the form of faeces. If performed in conjunction with vamana, it is typically administered a few days after the vamana treatment.

Basti

Basti is an enematherapy that purifies and nourishes the lower digestive tract by addressing vata imbalances. Excess vata toxins that have been brought back to the colon (site of origin for vata imbalances) by the purvakarma process are extracted downward via the introduction of a medicated enema. Since the vata dosha supports the transport of all toxins, basti is considered to be most important of all 5 therapies in panchakarma.

Nasya

Nasya involves inhaling medicated powders, liquids or vapour from herbal decoctions. Although nasya can address all the 3 doshas, it is particularly helpful in eliminating kapha-oriented problems. The nose is the gateway to the brain and to consciousness. Prana, or life-energy, enters the body through breath taken in through the nose. Nasya helps correct disorders of prana affecting the higher cerebral, sensory and motor functions.

Rakta Moksha

Rakta moksha therapy or bloodletting is used to eliminate toxins absorbed into the bloodstream through the gastrointestinal tract. The ultimate blood-purifying treatment, it is particularly useful for skin disorders. Traditionally, leeches are applied to the area of toxicity to suck out the poisonous blood. Nowadays a syringe is often used for the same purpose, although this is less effective than the traditional leech therapy.

Pashcaat Karma

Coming out of panchakarma, the physical body is depleted, and needs to rebuild strength and immunity through a nourishing diet, lifestyle therapies and rejuvenating therapies or rasayan. The treatment plan becomes much more prakruti-oriented or preventative. Its focus is on building ojas and reinvigorating the mind-body to function in a balanced dosha environment.

Ayurvedic Terms

agni	digestive fire
ama	bodily toxins, or undigested food matter
asana	yoga posture
Ayurveda	the 'science of life', India's ancient system of wellness
Brahma	creator of the universe; one of the 3 main gods in the Vedic tradition, he is believed to have spoken in the Rig Veda
chakras	energy centres of the body; the 7 major chakras are the top of the head, forehead, throat, heart, solar plexus, navel and lower abdomen, and the base of the spine

dinacharya	daily routine
Diwali	annual Hindu festival of lights that marks the Hindu New Year; Goddess Lakshmi is celebrated during this festival
dosha	an energetic force that is a combination of 2 of the 5 elements of nature and part of the make-up of each person; the 3 doshas are vata (air), pitta (fire) and kapha (water and earth)
River Ganga	holy river that runs through the northern Indians plains
jalneti	nasal cleansing practice (see pp. 82-83)
Lakshmi	goddess of wealth; she is the consort of Lord Vishnu and epitomizes the capacity of the kapha dosha: grounding, stability and prosperity
Lord Krishna	Hindu god, an incarnation of Vishnu who expounded the famous *Bhagavad Gita* (The Divine Song)
marma	vital points on the physical body where life energies are believed to be concentrated
ojas	the vitality, or essence, of the mind and body

panchakarma	classical Ayurvedic clinical detox regimen, involving complex procedures that require clinical supervision
Parvati	Vedic goddess of strength, she is the wife of Lord Shiva and epitomizes the capacity of the pitta dosha: strength and power
prakruti	natural state of balance; mind-body constitution
prana	breath, life-force
pranayama	yogic breathing practice
purvakarma	Ayurvedic massage, nutritional and body therapies that loosen toxins in the body so that they can be eliminated naturally
Radha	a shepherdess who was a devotee of Lord Krishna
rajas	the mental attributes of kingliness
rasayan	rejuvenating herbal concoctions that build and strengthen bones and tissues, and prevent aging; examples are ashwagandha, shatavari, brahmi and ghee

Rig Veda	the oldest of the 4 books of spiritual knowledge of India; Ayurveda was discussed in 3 books before being organized into its own system of healthcare
ritucharya	seasonal routine
Sanskrit	the language of ancient India and the ancient writings on Ayurveda
Saraswati	Vedic goddess of knowledge; consort of Lord Brahma, she epitomizes the capacity of the vata dosha: learning, creativity and art
sattwa	mental attribute of purity, balance
Shiva	destroyer of negativity, one of the three main gods in the Vedic tradition
svedana	heat therapy, one of the most common forms in the use of steam heat
tamas	mental attribute of dullness, inertia; toxic-minded
ubtan	a purifying legume-and-herb cleansing paste that is applied to the skin to purify the blood and circulatory system

vikruti	fluctuation or imbalance of physical and emotional elements which disrupts a person's natural wellbeing
Vishnu	the preserver of the universe, one of the 3 main gods in the Vedic tradition
yoga	a holistic Vedic science related to Ayurveda that improves health and vitality by harmonizing the mind, breath and body; Ayurvedic texts describe the components of yoga as ethical practices, rules or punctuality of daily routine, postures or physical exercises, breathing routines, sensory practices and meditation – postures and breathing are most predominantly practised as yoga today

References

Hora, Reenita Malhotra. 2005. *Inner Beauty*. San Francisco: Chronicle Books.

———. 2007. *Ayurveda: The Ancient Medicine of India*. San Francisco: Mandala Publishing.

Kulkarni, P. H. 1998. *Ayurveda Soundarayam*. Delhi: Sri Satguru Publications, a division of Indian Books Centre.

Nimbalkar, Sadashiv P. 1992. *Yoga for Health and Peace*. Bombay: Yoga Vidya Niketan.

Raichur, Pratima and Marian Cohn. 1997. *Absolute Beauty*. New York: HarperPerennial.

Rastogi, R. P. and B. N. Mehrotra. 1960–89. *Compendium of Indian Medicinal Plants*, 5 vols. New Delhi: National Institute of Science Communication.

Sharma, Ram Karan and Vaidya Bhagwan Dash. 2000. *Caraka Samhita*, 6th edn. Varanasi: Chaukhambha Sanskrit Series Office.

Vagabhata. 1999. *Ashtanga Hridayam*. Translated by a Board of Scholars. Delhi: Sri Satguru Publications, a division of Indian Books Centre.

Resources

Reenita Malhotra Hora, Ayurveda Clinician and Author
www.reenita.com

AYURVEDIC HERBS AND PRODUCTS

Baidyanath	www.baidyanath.com
Himalaya Herbal	www.himalayaherbals.com
Organic India	www.organicindia.co.in

AYURVEDIC BEAUTY PRODUCTS

Iraya	www.iraya.in
Omveda	www.omveda.com
Shahnaz Husain	www.shahnaz.in
Forest Essentials	www.forestessentialsindia.com
Khadi Natural	www.khadinatural.com

AYURVEDIC SPAS/PANCHA KARMA CENTRES

Kerala Ayurvedic Healthcare
www.keralaayurvedichealthcare.com/ayurveda/
ayurveda_centers.htm
VCC Ayurveda   www.vccayurveda.com
Vishwanath Panchakarma Ayurveda Centre
                      www.panchkarma.org
Arya Vaidya Shala   http://aryavaidyasala.com
Jiva Ayurveda   www.jiva.com

YOGA/AYURVEDA CENTRES

Krishnamacharya Centre
                      www.kym.org
Satyananda Yoga Mandiram
                      www.satyanandayogacenter.com
Sivananda Yoga Vedanta Centre
                      www.sivananda.org/trivandrum
Parmarth Niketan   www.parmarth.com

AYURVEDA RETREATS

New Ideal Panchakarma Centre
                      www.panchakarmakerala.com
Soukya   www.soukya.com

Kandamkulathy AyurSoukhyam Ayurvedic Resort
www.ayursoukhyam.com
Kalarikovilakom www.cghearth.com

Acknowledgements

This book has been a labour of love. Hopefully it will be as inspiring to read as it was to write.

My thanks go to: Anjali Joshi, our family yoga guru, for supporting my interest in pursuing the study of yoga, Ayurveda and the Vedic sciences; Kathryn Keller, my colleague at the Institute of Health and Healing in San Francisco, who consulted on the yoga section of this book; Priya Doraswamy, my agent, who encouraged me to take all the steps to bring this project to fruition; and at Pan Macmillan India, Saugata Mukherjee, my publisher, for taking a chance on this book and Pallavi Narayan, my editor, for her tireless effort in editing and re-editing the manuscript.

I thank Gopal Krishan Vij, my late grandfather, who first taught me the secrets of staying forever young, and encouraged me to write down everything I wanted to say to the world; Neeraj Hora, who encourages me to look for beauty in situations that might not outwardly appear beautiful; Veena and Rajinder Malhotra, who have always believed in me; Ilya Devi and Arya Vir Hora, who inspire me to maximize ojas every day; and Sushma Hora, who honed my fascination for the healing properties of medicinal plants.

All teachers, practitioners, and missionaries of Ayurveda – it is your dedication that inspires people to seek out this life-changing philosophy in the first place.

All you folks interested in Ayurveda, I hope that you share this wellness philosophy with others.